Call Of The Jungle

How a Camping-Hating City-Slicker Mum
Survived an Ultra Endurance Race through the
Amazon Jungle

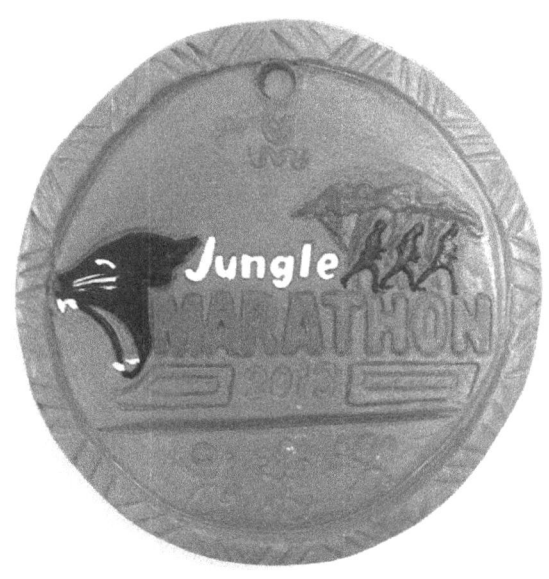

By Amanda Barlow

Copyright © 2014 Amanda Barlow

All rights reserved.

Photography: Alexander Beer Photography
Cover: Alex Dumitru – Image Trance

ISBN: 978-0-646-91882-2

DISCLAIMER

This book depicts the author's own experiences while competing in the Jungle Marathon 2013 and has been written to give the reader an insight into the extreme conditions and physical demands placed on competitors in the multi-day ultra-endurance event in the Amazon Jungle. The author is not an authority on ultra-endurance racing and is not expressing advice on how to compete in one, merely relaying an account of her own participation in the event. It is not a recommendation to participate in the Jungle Marathon and it must be stressed that anyone interested in competing in this ultra-endurance event must be well trained and physically fit to endure the extreme conditions that will be encountered. While every safeguard is taken to minimize the risk of harm to competitors it is impossible to predict every potential outcome and runners agree to run at their own risk and that they are medically fit to do so.

Dedicated to Chris, Alex and Becky.

"May you always have an open mind and adventurous spirit."

CONTENTS

	ACKNOWLEDGMENTS	i
	INTRODUCTION	ix
1	PREPARING FOR THE JUNGLE MARATHON	11
2	TRAVELLING TO BRAZIL	17
3	ACCLIMATIZING IN THE JUNGLE	25
4	THE BASE CAMP	32
5	RACE DAY – STAGE 1	72
6	RACE DAY – STAGE 2	105
7	RACE DAY – STAGE 3	126
8	RACE DAY – STAGE 4	150
9	RACE DAY – STAGE 5	194
10	RACE DAY – STAGE 6	220
11	THE PRESENTATION DINNER	230
12	JUNGLE MARATHON CONCLUSION	236
	EPILOGUE	241
	JUNGLE MARATHON RACE RESULTS	242
	ABOUT THE AUTHOR	247

A portion of the proceeds from the sale of this book goes towards the Fiona Forrest Charity Fund for Elisama Orphanage, Indonesia.

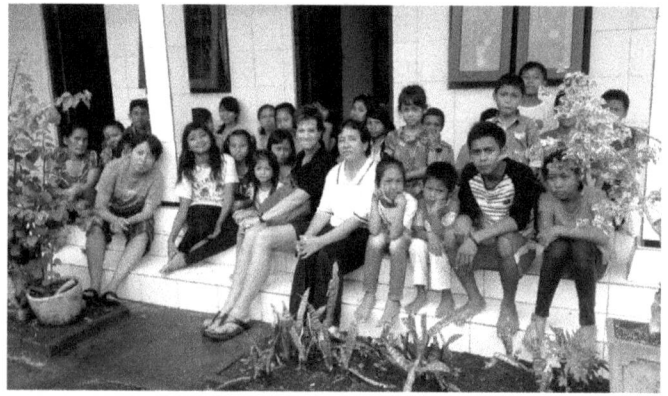

While I am living my privileged life to the fullest Fiona Forrest is selflessly helping to make the world a better place for those less privileged. I hope the sales of this book help contribute to your amazing efforts.

ACKNOWLEDGMENTS

An event like the Jungle Marathon could never exist without the combined effort of many people from all around the world. This is truly an international smorgasbord of the world's most enthusiastic runners, medics, volunteers, photographers and local hosts who, despite a language barrier, come together with the help of event sponsors UVU and Event Rate, to make this event a most remarkable experience.

A special thank-you to Gustavo Rodrigues, who is not only a remarkable ultra-endurance athlete but also a representative for ICMBio, the government body that oversees the preservation of the Tapajos National Forest and liaises with the race director to enable competitors to experience the true beauty of the Amazon Jungle.

I'm sure I speak on behalf of all the competitors in thanking the local village people who played hosts to us along our journey through the Amazon Jungle and supplied us with a place to hang our hammocks at the end of the exhausting days. They also gave up their time to oversee the distribution of drinking water and gave us a taste of the real Amazon Jungle that tourists never get to experience.

The medical team did a fantastic job of attending to everyone's needs under the leadership of the Jungle Marathon's emergency care specialists Jeremy Joslin and Vicky Kypta. The 16-strong fun-loving, yet truly professional, team never failed to lift our spirits at the checkpoints with their smiling faces and eagerness to help in any way they could. The additional help from ultra-endurance athlete, and author of "Fixing Your Feet," John Vonhof at the base camps, topped off the world-class group of race medics. I'm sure he would have got some excellent material for another book after treating so many disgusting feet throughout the course of the race. No man should have to experience that much toe jam but he did it with the grace and eloquence of a true ultra runner!

Many thanks also to the spirited race volunteers who provided help and support at the checkpoints. The international volunteer crew added to the atmosphere of the event and it was great to have met you all.

Critical to the success of the event was the help of all the local people involved in race organizing under the guidance of the race director. Unfortunately the language barrier meant that I was limited to a wave or thumbs up gesture to convey my appreciation but this did not make it any less sincere. This group also included the Brazilian Bombeiros (military firemen) who provided their experience and expertise in the jungle environment, and also the support of Simone, the race director's assistant. Bridging the cultural divide to get the job done may not have been successful *all* of the time but every great adventure has it's share of unplanned situations which make it all the more memorable.

A special acknowledgement goes out to all the competitors who participated in the 2013 Jungle Marathon and added their own personality to the unique event. The camaraderie enjoyed by so many like-minded people under such extraordinary conditions is what makes a trip like this so rewarding. Regardless of where you come in the final results table it is the experience that you remember for a lifetime. A very special thanks to Karen, Danielle, Jason and Ed who helped me survive stages 2 and 3 and provided much needed pacesetting and a distraction from my pain with their conversation. I'm sorry if I slowed you down! My one regret is that I didn't spend more time getting to know more of the competitors, due to either the language barrier or the fact that I barely had the energy to open my mouth at the end of the race days. It was a pleasure to have been in the company of such amazing athletes and you all well and truly earned, and deserved, your medals.

Although I will always carry the memories of the race with me in my mind, it is an added bonus to have photographs of me in this remarkable environment as a permanent record of how incredibly brave – or how recklessly stupid – I can be when I put my mind to it! A big shout out to the film crew from TV Globo's Planeta Extremo who extended their Brazilian hospitality to me in Alter do Chao and then screamed encouragement at me from the "press gallery" through the jungle swamps. Your enthusiasm was contagious and brought a smile to my face at times when I was ready to cry like a girl and yell, "this is too hard!"

An extra special thank-you goes to the official race photographer, Alexander Beer, for capturing the essence of the Jungle Marathon through the lens of his camera. The only way he could get the special shots, like the one on the cover of this book, was by being in the swamps himself and exposing himself to the same risks as the competitors. Fellow photographer Nigel Swan was equally as dedicated in capturing the best shots possible in the formidable terrain.

I have kept the greatest acknowledgement until last so

it's obvious to all reading this just how much work goes into holding an event like the Jungle Marathon and how many people have to be organized to make it all happen. The race director, Shirley Thompson, has made possible arguably the world's most extreme ultra-endurance race, despite the logistical nightmares that accompany organizing it in one of the harshest and most remote locations on the planet. The 9th running of the Jungle Marathon would prove to be the most challenging yet for Shirley, with a medical emergency of her own to contend with after a close encounter with the local wildlife, and then a dramatic twist to the end of the marathon stage that would threaten not only the final stages of the 2013 event but could also cast a shadow over the future of the Jungle Marathon. I have no doubt Shirley will overcome the hurdles and continue to provide a world-class event for ultra-endurance athletes from all around the world who are looking for the ultimate challenge. I would never have guessed at the time of my serendipitous introduction to Shirley when we were paired up as tent buddies during the Antarctic Ice Marathon, that I would be participating in an ultra-endurance race through the Amazon Jungle only 12 months later. Thanks Shirley for the adventure of a lifetime!

******

My story would never have got out of my head if it wasn't for the creative genius of Steve and Pam Brossman. Pam's Digital Boost Marketing course helped me make the giant leap from writer to published author and enable me to turn my running adventure into a published book that can be shared with everyone. I'm grateful for the encouragement, passion and depth of knowledge you both provided to help make this book happen.

I would also like to thank my diligent proof reader and editor, Mike Kenny, who re-affirmed what I had already suspected – that I have forgotten nearly everything I learnt in high school English grammar lessons!

Final edits from Roslyn Budd were greatly appreciated also.

A special thanks also to Alex Dumitru of Imagetrance.com for designing the book cover and capturing the essence of the Jungle Marathon in his amazing design.

CALL OF THE JUNGLE

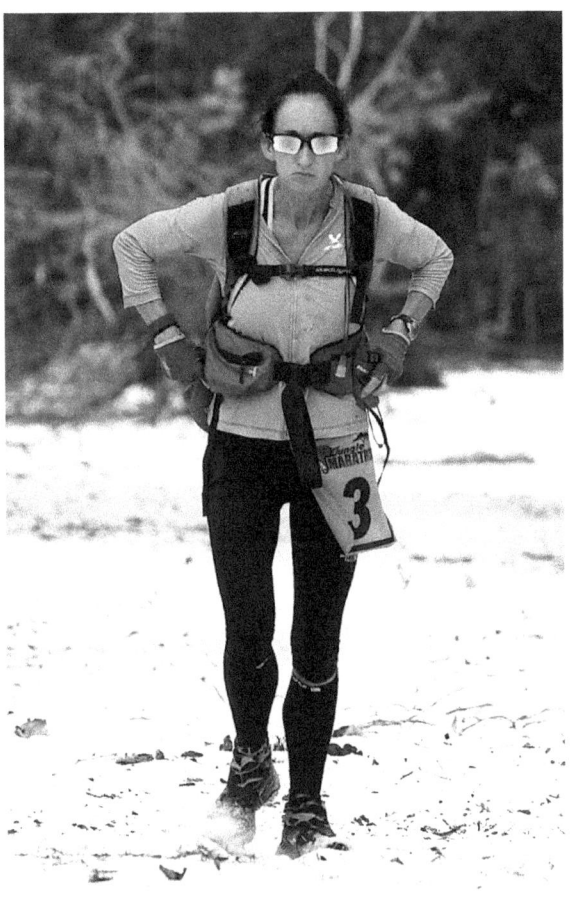

"That which doesn't kill us makes us stronger."
- *Friedrich Nietzsche*

CALL OF THE JUNGLE

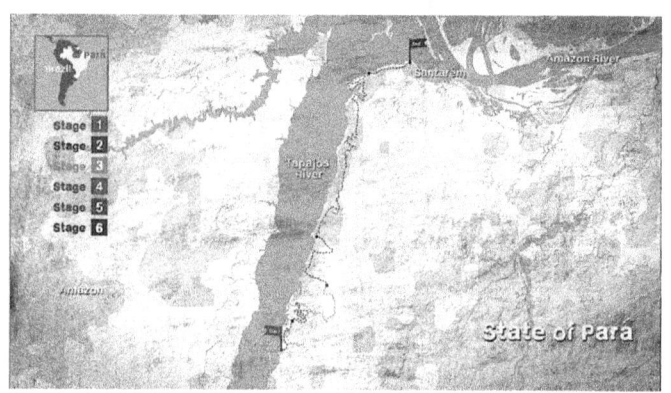

INTRODUCTION

The Jungle Marathon is a 254km multi-stage, unsupported ultra-endurance race through the heart of the Amazon Jungle. The full 254km event consists of 6 stages run over 7 days but there are also two shorter options; a 127km 4-stage event over 4 consecutive days and a 1 day stand-alone 42km marathon event, which doubles as the 4th stage of the 4-stage event, for those not interested in doing the multi-day events.

This race has been voted by CNN as the toughest endurance race in the world and the testimonials from athletes who have completed it leave no doubt that the unforgiving and hostile environment of the Amazon Jungle is the ultimate endurance athletes challenge.

The adventure begins in Alter do Chao in northern Brazil, on the banks of the Tapajos River. The race competitors and support crew travel by riverboat up the Tapajos River to a base camp at Prainha. There, they spend 2 days and nights camping in the jungle while acclimatizing and being briefed on what is to come. All competitors must be self-sufficient for the 2 days at the base camp and the 7 days of their race. The only thing provided by the organizers is cold and hot water for drinking and meals. All of your equipment, including food, is to be carried on your back for the duration of the race, which provides the ultimate challenge of endurance. Your backpack contains compulsory items such as a hammock, fly net, rain sheet, medical and survival supplies, food, 2.5 litres of water carrying capacity, along with any personal requirements such as clothes, toiletries, camera, etc.

The route consists of river and swamp crossings in primary jungle, very steep climbs and descents, tracks through deep jungle areas where jaguars roam freely, and beautiful fluvial beaches that separate the Amazonian waters from the dense jungle canopy. The terrain is both stunningly beautiful and soul-destroying in its extremeness.

The extreme heat and humidity can have devastating effects on unacclimatized athletes and many fall victim to this every year. It's impossible to tell who may be affected but the sure thing is that every year *someone* will be affected!

Chapter 1

PREPARING FOR THE JUNGLE MARATHON

Why The Jungle Marathon?

While researching for the Antarctic Ice Marathon in 2012 I came across a website for the Jungle Marathon, which shares a mutual sponsor (UVU) with the Ice Marathon. I remember reading the details of the event and thinking at the time there is no way in the world I would ever do anything that tough. The website gave graphic details of several days running through the Amazon Jungle, swimming through piranha-infested rivers, negotiating kilometer-long stream descents, trudging through swamps in thigh-deep mud, countless near-vertical hill climbs, and all of this while sleeping in hammocks at campsites with no facilities whatsoever at the end of each day and surrounded by some of the deadliest animals and insects the world can throw at you. That's insane!!

Well, fast forward to November 2012 when I had just landed at the glacial campsite for the Antarctic Ice Marathon and had been allocated my 2-man tent with a pre-selected "tent buddy" by the name of Shirley Thompson – who just happens to be the creator and race director of the Jungle Marathon!

Needless to say, Shirley had a captive audience of about 50 crazy marathoners who would undoubtedly be looking for their next fix of extreme marathoning to do in some far-flung corner of the world. There's no doubt that after completing the Antarctic Ice Marathon you've set the marathon experience bar pretty high and no normal run-of-the-mill marathon is going to satisfy you any more.

After 5 days of sitting around a single communal dining tent and talking about marathons it was inevitable that Shirley would entice everyone with the challenge of competing in the world's toughest endurance race. At the time I was still basking in the glory of being one of the privileged few to have run a marathon on the most remote continent in the world and was soaking up the surreal atmosphere and unique scenery of the Union Glacier campsite. Also, I was already registered to run the Boston Marathon in April 2013 so I thought my future running challenges were already taken care of.

Within weeks of getting home and the post-marathon euphoria a fading memory, my new Facebook friends from the Antarctica trip started posting updates about doing the Jungle Marathon. All it took was seeing one person say they had registered and I was hooked. Somehow the Jungle Marathon had just gone from being this insane event that no one in their right mind would attempt, to an exciting adventure that I just had to be a part of. How that change of mind occurred I will never know!

From the moment I registered and paid my first deposit for the Jungle Marathon, my life revolved around a commitment that was far removed from anything I had ever done before. With no past experience to compare it to, I had to hope that my baseline fitness would get me through the event. It seemed that I had now raised the "bar" a notch higher and the marathons I would do leading up to the Jungle Marathon were to be training runs instead of the individual goals they had once been.

Training for the Jungle Marathon

When the day finally came to start the long trip over to Alter do Chao, where our boat was to depart to take us to the jungle camp where we would start our multi-day event, I thought I was well prepared for what lay ahead of me but boy, was I to be proven wrong in the days ahead!

Six weeks earlier, after already completing three road marathons throughout the year (Hobart, Boston and Brisbane), I competed in what I thought would have given me a good conditioning training run for the Jungle Marathon, by doing the Lamington Eco Challenge, in South East Queensland, Australia, which consisted of back-to-back trail marathons on two consecutive days. I thought running this grueling 42km event, down and back up the side of a mountain, not just once but twice over two consecutive days, wearing the backpack I would be using in the Jungle Marathon loaded with 2 litres of water, would be a good simulation of what I could expect in the jungle.

After surviving the Eco Challenge and then running the Sydney Marathon (the sixth marathon for the year) just 10 days before departing for Brazil, I was feeling very comforted by the fact that I was injury-free and had lots of running miles under my belt.

Although I had done nearly all of my training runs on a treadmill and hadn't done the recommended training in wet runners, I still felt that the five road and two trail marathons I'd completed in the previous 10 months would give me the base fitness to survive in the jungle. I spend half of the year working in the tropics, so I was pretty sure the hot weather and humidity wouldn't bother me, and my socks are always ringing wet (literally!) when I finish my morning training sessions so I thought my feet would probably be OK in the jungle conditions. I had also never suffered from blisters or toenail problems, ever, in any of my previous marathon runs, and I had been doing up to 7 marathons a year over the previous 2 years, so I was quietly confident that my feet would hold up to the task.

With departure day drawing closer I began to dread the five flights I would have to endure to get to the start location and was slightly concerned about the possibility of my luggage getting lost during one of the airport transfers. As I had never done an ultra distance event before, let alone one in the jungle, I really had no clue as to what things I would need, so I prepared clothes and gear for all contingencies. There were compulsory items that we had to take, like a hammock, a medical kit, and enough food to be self-sufficient in the jungle for 9 days, in addition to the race clothing that we would need to survive the harsh and dangerous conditions we were going to be facing.

The Final Checks

My last night at home was spent packing all of my gear and crosschecking against my list of compulsory race items one last time to ensure that I had everything I needed. Apart from food, clothing and personal items, there were many compulsory items we had to carry with us including: insect repellent, a compass, safety pins, a knife, a medical kit including salt tablets, pain killers, disinfectant, tape, bandages etc., a torch and spare batteries, waterproof matches or a lighter, water-purifying tablets for at least 10 litres, an emergency whistle and two light sticks. I also had a bag full of dehydrated meals and snacks that I divided up into daily rations that I thought would cover my nutrition needs. My experience with marathons told me that you have very specific needs when performing endurance events and even though you know what your body needs after a long sustained event, your stomach generally has other ideas! I just wanted to make sure I had more than enough food to cover any contingencies, given that we wouldn't be able to buy anything once we got into the jungle.

While I was checking and packing all of my gear, my son was busy Google-searching dangerous Amazon Jungle animals and came across the famed "bullet ant", which he excitedly read out to me as having the most painful bite of any insect in the world. He assured me it was found in the area of the Amazon Jungle that I would be spending nine days camping in and he delighted in reading out aloud the horrifying statistics of this infamous insect. The only comforting fact seemed to be that it was not poisonous, just very painful. Well if it can't kill me then I don't really have to worry too much about it, I thought. I had already resigned myself to the fact that I was sure to get bites and stings out there, so determined I'd just have to put up with the discomfort and push on regardless. It was certainly too late to start worrying about being bitten by an ant, so I finished my packing and lay down in my comfy bed, knowing it would be the last time for a couple of weeks that I would enjoy such a luxury.

Chapter 2

TRAVELLING TO BRAZIL

My trip started with my son driving me for 60 minutes from the Gold Coast to Brisbane and dropping me off at the airport. My job has me working away, flying in and out of Brisbane Airport every 4 weeks, and I also make frequent trips away between working, so it's not uncommon for my son to be dropping me off at the airport.

This time was different though. For the first time ever he came around to the curb and as he was coming towards me, said: "I better give you a hug…you never know…". It was at this point I started to wonder if I was underestimating the challenges of the event I was about to take part in?? And just to drive the point home even further, as he stepped back into the car he called back to me and said: "I sort of hope you get bitten by a bullet ant so you can tell me what it was like!", and with those parting words I entered the controlled environment of the Brisbane International Airport, which would be the starting point for my journey through the sterile world of airports and airplanes until I popped back out into the real world again in the tropical air of the Amazon Jungle two days later.

My trip saw me changing flights in Sydney, Santiago

(Chile), Sao Paulo (southeastern Brazil), and Belem (northern Brazil) before finally arriving at Santarem, located in central northern Brazil. Santarem Airport was very small, requiring we disembark from the plane onto the tarmac and then walk along the back of the terminal building and into the arrivals lounge. As the other passengers slowly filled up the room I couldn't help but wonder if any of these people were "Jungle Marathoners". I glanced around the room at all the people and checked for signs of ultra-endurance athletes but everyone just looked like your average traveller, however, so did I. Dressed in comfortable travel clothes I looked more like the 53-year-old mother of three that I really am, rather than an athlete about to embark on an epic journey through the Amazon Jungle!

With all the different flights I had been on I was very concerned about the possibility of my bags not arriving at the same time as me, so I wasn't ready to relax just yet. I had carried the most essential items I would need to be able to participate in the Jungle Marathon in a bag small enough to be carried as cabin luggage, just in case a baggage mishap occurred. When you have trained so hard and invested so much money leading up to an event, you are acutely aware that so many things that are out of your control can de-rail your best efforts.

Leading up to the day of your departure your biggest fear is developing an injury or illness that can prevent you from training. Once you get to the airport, the fear of injury is overtaken by the fear of one or more of the many flights being delayed or cancelled, which is why I like to try and arrive at my destination at least one or two days ahead of the actual event date. Finally, when you get there, you cross your fingers and pray to the baggage Gods that all of your bags arrive at the same time you do.

I waited at 01:15am for the baggage carousel to start up, going through a mental check of the preparations I had completed over the past several months to be able to get to where I was now standing. To be injury-free after already running several marathons in the past 10 months was a comforting thought. To have travelled half way around the world, have all of my flights successfully connecting and to have the most essential items for the event still with me was one more weight off my shoulders. To my surprise, once the carousel finally came to life, my bags were some of the first to appear through the hatch. I couldn't believe my luck! Now there remained just one further hurdle – finding a taxi at 01:30am to take me to Alter do Chao, a small town 33km west of Santarem, where we were to board the riverboat that would take us to the base camp.

I followed the crowd out of the small arrivals room into the pick-up area in front of the terminal building and was relieved to see a row of taxis lined up waiting for passengers. Although the place was bustling with people now, I could sense that within a very short period of time everyone would have scurried away to find a comfortable bed to crash in, leaving the area like a deserted ghost town. I was feeling safe surrounded by a busy hub of weary travellers and didn't like the thought of being left on my own in the still of the night, so I raced to the first taxi in the line and in Portuguese-accented English tried to explain where I wanted to go.

I have no idea why English-speaking people trying to converse in a foreign language, from which they don't know a single word, attempt to speak with an accent, as if the foreigner is going to understand English words when they're pronounced differently. But I still find myself doing it, and cringe when I hear it roll out of my mouth! How I envy people who are multi-lingual. It's at moments like this that I can't help but marvel at the millions of people around the world, many from less affluent societies than the one I come from, who struggle to learn English as a second language so they can communicate with ignorant English-speaking natives who visit their country but are too lazy to learn the local language. However, Brazil doesn't seem to be one of those countries where the locals adopt English, as no-one seems to speak it.

As I prepared to ask the taxi driver if he could take me to the Beloalter Hotel in Alter do Chao, and how much it would cost me, I was hoping that the hotel and town names were written the same in both English and Portuguese so the hotel reservation I printed out could act as my interpreter. I hoped I could just show him the piece of paper and he would know straight away where I wanted to go. I desperately wanted to see his face light up and smile at me in understanding, such that he knew what I wanted without having to actually try and say anything. But no, all I received was a vacant, perplexed look and some rambling in a language that may as well have been Swahili! Oh no, now it meant I would have to try and talk in Portuguese-accented English.... the shame!!

Fortunately my embarrassingly shameful pronunciation of Alter do Chao managed to register with him, after pointing to the name of the hotel on my reservation itinerary, and his face finally started to show a glimpse of recognition. Phew! The next challenge to conquer was finding out how much the ride would cost. I suspected any non-Portuguese speaking tourist would be fair game for being ripped off and I didn't want to find out when I got to my destination in the sleepy little village of Alter do Chao at 2am that he was demanding a ridiculously high fare. So in a stupid, embarrassing accent I asked: "how many Real?" and to my travel-weary delight he responded by writing down the number 90 on a notepad. Finally we were on the same page!

Shirley, the Jungle Marathon race director, had told me the cab fare from Santarem Airport to Alter do Chao would cost around R$100 so I was happy that the driver wasn't trying to rip me off and I gave him a thumbs up and a nod to indicate that I was happy with his fare. With that we pulled away from the curb and started the trip to a place even smaller than the one I had flown in to.

It was only a matter of minutes before we were out of the city streetlights and on a dark, narrow two-lane sealed road winding through lush rainforest. During the 30-minute drive to Alter do Chao we only saw a few other cars on the road, with their approaching headlights giving me minor relief in knowing that I wasn't the only person out in the middle of nowhere in the middle of the night.

As tired as I was, I still found it hard to relax and, although each set of approaching headlights would at first make me feel a bit more at ease, I would quickly turn my thoughts around to thinking that maybe the people in the approaching car could be opportunistic jungle rebel fighters who think that anyone stupid enough to be on a dark jungle road at this ridiculous time of the night was fair game to be robbed or kidnapped for the greater good of their cause.

After all, the Australian Department of Foreign Affairs and Trade (DFAT) was advising travelers to exercise a high degree of caution in Brazil because of the high levels of serious and violent crimes such as muggings, armed robbery, kidnappings and sexual assault. Admittedly, they say this is especially of concern in the big cities however, I couldn't help thinking about a recent news article I had read about a small town somewhere in northern Brazil where a football referee was stoned to death and then beheaded by the players and spectators of a game he was overseeing in retaliation for having stabbed a player to death because he refused to leave the field when told to. My sixth sense was hauntingly reminding me that I was alone, in the middle of the night, on a dark and lonely jungle road in a foreign country where extreme violence was an accepted part of life.

We finally arrived at the sleeping town of Alter do Chao and drove through the pot-holed streets in the wee hours of the morning before pulling into the grounds of the hotel. I was relieved to see the name of the hotel above the main entrance, confirming I was at the correct destination, but the hotel was in darkness and I started imagining myself sleeping on the steps of the reception office waiting for them to open. To my surprise though, the taxi driver set about finding someone to let me in and waited until my reservation had been confirmed before departing. Despite the fact the hotel manager didn't speak any English, the check-in process went without a hitch and I was soon being guided down the tropical garden path to my room - I was finally on my way to a bed!

The Beloalter Hotel in Alter do Chao is set amongst beautiful green rainforest grounds on the banks of the

Lago Verde (Green Lake). The room was basic but comfortable and clean, with a working air conditioner and a good shower, so I was pleasantly relieved that I still had two nights in a comfortable hotel before facing several nights of roughing it in the jungle.

The room also seemed to be free of any mosquitoes, which was a relief as I was now in malaria territory and although I had started taking anti-malarial tablets two days before leaving home, it seems these are not always a guarantee against contracting the disease. I had purchased a super-strong 80% DEET insect repellent from the travel doctor before leaving home but really didn't want to have to use it if at all possible because it was very thick, sticky and smelly. The only other essential immunization for travelling to the Amazon Jungle was for Yellow Fever but I had already had one of those shots a couple of years earlier when I travelled to Tanzania to do the Kilimanjaro Marathon. As they last for 5 years there was no need for me to have it again.

After unpacking my toiletries I had a shower and looked forward to sleeping in a comfortable bed, relieved at the thought of not having to do any travelling for another couple of days. The next day was a free day to do what I wanted and acclimatize to the tropical weather, so I could sleep in for as long as I wanted.

Arriving at my destination so late in the night meant I would probably not suffer from jet lag. I knew I was exhausted enough to fall asleep for several hours so it would be just like a normal night's sleep. I had arrived a day and a half early just to make sure though, aside from allowing time for any possible baggage loss during the many legs of the trip.

For the first time in two days and two nights I felt like I could finally relax – my flights were all on schedule and got me to where I had to be 2 days early, my bags all arrived at the same time, I got to my hotel safely *and* my hotel reservation was confirmed and a room prepared for me. I felt like I could finally let my guard down and I had done everything possible to get me safely to the start of the Jungle Marathon.

Everything from here on was in the hands of the race director and all that was left to do now was to settle into "jungle time" and forget about schedules and routines for the next 9 days. After a quick shower, the feel of my clean skin against the crisp hotel bed sheets had a tranquilizing effect on my mind and my body and I knew my glorious long-awaited sleep would only be moments away.

Chapter 3

ACCLIMATIZING IN THE JUNGLE

Alter do Chao

Alter do Chao is located 33km west of the Amazon port city of Santarem, along one of the only roads in the northern Brazilian state of Para. The small village is located on the Tapajos River and next to Lago Verde. It is best known for a picturesque white sand island, known as Ilha do Amor (Island of Love), which lies opposite the village and between the two bodies of water. As the Amazon River water level recedes in summer the sand bank grows and the locals take advantage of the idyllic white sand and aqua-colored water by setting up bars and providing water sport activities for the tourists who flock to the area.

While I definitely wanted to check out the Ilha do Amor, I still had two full days in Alter do Chao so decided there was no rush to go beyond the serene boundaries of the Beloalter Hotel for the first morning. After a glorious non-interrupted recovery sleep, my only priority was to get to the complimentary buffet breakfast before it closed.

The dining area was out on a large deck to the rear of the reception building and looked out over the lush rainforest gardens of the hotel grounds. While most of the food looked quite foreign to me, I managed to fill myself up on boiled eggs, toast and an assortment of local fruits.

It was going to be a hot day and the humidity was already suffocatingly high but it wasn't anything that I wasn't already accustomed to. Once you've accepted the fact that your skin is going to stay damp all day and your hair go all frizzy and unmanageable, you're alright!

I took my laptop to breakfast with me hoping I could get a Wi-Fi connection. Although I couldn't get one in the dining area, it was possible to pick it up in the reception lounge, so after finishing eating I made myself comfortable in a corner chair and checked my emails and Facebook.

I'm not sure if it's a good thing or bad thing that you can now stay in touch and communicate in real time from even the most remote parts of the world. It has a comfort value when you are travelling alone. Checking into Facebook and reading what your friends were doing while you were off the grid for two days travelling to the other side of the world, makes you feel like you're only a keystroke away from company if you need it. The nine days I would be spending in the jungle would be communication-free so I thought I might as well stay in touch with everyone while I could.

By late morning it was getting very warm so I thought I'd go down to the hotel pool. At the back of the dining area there was a bar facility leading out onto the pool. The pool was only small, about 10-15m long, but looked very inviting in the tropical heat and humidity. The water temperature was about 30°C which was exactly how I like it – no freezing shock to the body when you jump in, just a cooling relief on your clammy hot skin.

While lounging around the pool area I met up with a

group of Brazilians who were also doing the Jungle Marathon. Out of the several people in the group, only two of them were competing and the others were a film crew who were going to record the whole event. The two runners were journalists who were doing the event as part of a series of TV programs on extreme sports. Fortunately these people spoke some English and they invited me to join them as they prepared for an afternoon BBQ down in a shady area near the bank of the Lago Verde, which was about 50m further on from the pool area.

Later in the afternoon we were joined by Shirley Thompson, the race director, and while chatting about the race with her I became horrifyingly stunned by the fact, that I had somehow misinterpreted in all the race logistics emails - the race was "*fully* self-supported", which meant that each competitor had to carry *everything* they would need for the duration of the entire race.

For me, as I had naively registered to do the full 254km event, it meant I would have to carry all of my gear for 7 days of racing on my back - not just a small back pack with 2.5 litres of water and the snacks I would need for the individual stages each day, but everything I would need for the entire week – including a hammock with fly net and rain sheet, food for 7 days, 2.5 litres of water, full medical kit, clothes, personal items, toiletries – EVERYTHING!! The only thing that would be provided was hot water to add to dehydrated food pouches or cold water – nothing else.

For some unknown reason I just assumed that all of our camp supplies, like hammock, spare clothes, toiletries, bedding (like the nice little pillow I had for my hammock and the small sleeping bag in case it got cool over night) and the few changes of clean T-shirts and shorts, etc., were going to be transported to the next campsite for us each day by the race support crew. How could I have missed this fundamental key point???

Everyone else seemed to know this fact but me! My total lack of experience in ultra-endurance marathons had now just struck its first blow. After spending about 15 minutes freaking out and then processing the thought of how I was going to manage the unexpected change to my race plan, I decided not to let this put me off achieving my goal of completing the Jungle Marathon. I would just have to accept the fact I would have to forget about running the entire race and instead just walk most of the way, which was a compromise I was happy to make. Shirley offered to lend me a bigger backpack (a 25-litre one instead of the 20-litre one that I had) that would fit all the extra gear in it, so I took her up on the offer and started to relax again, thinking that I would still be up for the task of completing the 7-day event.

I spent that evening trying to figure out how I was going to fit everything I needed for the 7 days of racing into that small backpack. It was becoming glaringly obvious that I had brought along about five times more gear than I would need – *or be able to carry* – so I had to make the decision on what would be essential and what could be left behind on the boat. As I wouldn't get the pack from Shirley until we left for the jungle I still wasn't exactly sure how much stuff I could actually fit into a 25-litre backpack, but knew it wouldn't be anywhere near what I knew I'd need.

I went to bed feeling a bit annoyed that I had brought so much stuff with me that I'd now have to carry around until the start of the race. I tried not to let it bother me too much though because I wanted to enjoy my last night of sleeping on a comfortable bed in an air-conditioned room before setting out for the jungle base camp the following evening. After that, it would just be a hammock strung between two trees for a week.

Ilha do Amor

After filling up on the buffet breakfast the next morning I ventured out of the grounds of the Beloalter Hotel and went for a walk to the village centre, which was about 2km from the hotel. The mid-morning sun was already very hot and, thanks to the tropical humidity, sweat was drenching my skin within minutes of starting the walk.

After wandering through the old pot-holed streets, I was surprised when I came to the end of a street and found the Ilha do Amor stretching out across the water like a sliver of paradise in the oppressive jungle heat. It was like the reverse of a lush oasis in a sandy desert. Instead, it was a sandy oasis in a thick jungle with the sun glistening on the turquoise water and reflecting brightly off the fine white sand, making it look more like a Caribbean island than a riverbank a thousand kilometers inland from the sea.

I walked along the riverbank walkway and came to the village Waste, which is where all the Jungle Marathoners were to meet up later that day in preparation for departure by riverboat at approximately 11pm. The Square was surrounded by tourist shops, bars and café's and had a lively atmosphere about it. It felt like you were in some coastal beach resort town, rather than a village in the middle of the Amazon Jungle, with the mesmerizing "Island of Love" front and center stage, masquerading as an idyllic holiday destination rather than the simple spit of sand on the Tapajos River that it was.

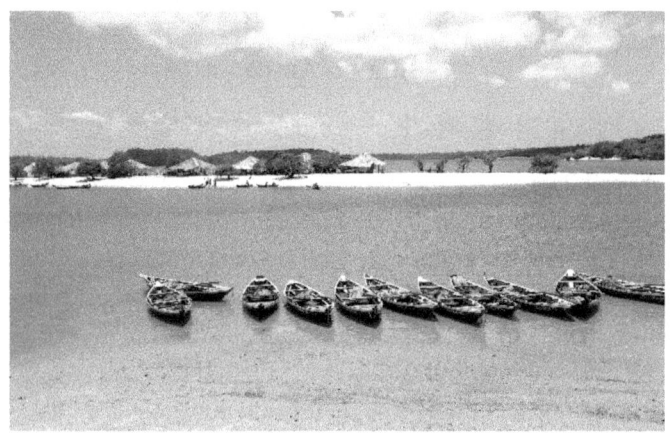

There were a dozen canoes lined up along the riverbank ready to ferry tourists over the 100m channel that separated the Tapajos River from the Lago Verde, so they could get to the Ilha do Amour without having to risk being nibbled by piranhas. The sandbar island had a line of several thatched-roofed open-air bars that served food and drinks to the people sitting at the tables laid out on the sand.

After walking the length of the village shorelines I headed back to the hotel, met up with the film crew again at the

BBQ area near the Lago Verde shore and joined them for lunch. I was concerned about how I was going to get all of my bags down to the village Square, suspecting that the village wasn't big enough to support a taxi service, so was relieved when the crew said they would have enough room in their vehicles to be able to carry me, and all of my bags, down to the meeting point later in the afternoon.

Chapter 4

THE BASE CAMP

Leaving For The Jungle

The time came for us all to meet at the village Square in Alter do Chao, where we would board the boat that would take us up the Tapajos River to our base camp. By the time I arrived late in the afternoon, the Square was already full of backpacking Jungle Marathoners who had travelled from numerous countries all around the world.

The last newsletter we received stated there were going to be 76 competitors between the 42km, 127km and 254km events, twelve of these being females, with runners coming from Argentina, Austria, Australia, Brazil, China, Chile, England, Germany, Greece, Japan, Italy, Norway, New Zealand, Netherlands, Serbia, Venezuela, Wales, South Africa, Slovenia, Spain, Scotland and the USA.

Looking around at the luggage most of the other runners were carrying, I began to feel very embarrassed by the excessive amount of gear I was lugging around. I had one large case just full of camp food, another full of camping supplies and another smaller one with clothes and toiletries in it. Most competitors seemed to have one large backpack and a smaller race pack, but on further investigation I began to find a few others with over-sized bags and carrying equally as much gear as me, so I tried to relax and hope that I didn't look too conspicuous as an ill-prepared ultra jungle marathoner.

The Portuguese film crew started interviewing some of the competitors, with portable mini flood lights illuminating the area in the fading light of early evening. With most of the competitors probably in the Square now, the atmosphere was starting to get very lively with the realization that the adventure was about to get under way.

The language barrier seemed to naturally segregate the crowd into different nationalities and I followed suit by introducing myself to the first English-speaking person I came across.

Becky was a doctor from the UK and was part of the large medical team that would be accompanying us into the jungle. Running in such a harsh environment meant the competitors could be faced with many possible threats that they wouldn't normally be exposed to during most other events around the world. Not only would people likely be inflicted with the annoying, but not generally life-threatening, feet blisters and body chaffing but they also risked more serious complaints like dehydration and heat stress, infections from skin wounds and insect bites or stings, through to life-threatening venomous animal bites. In previous years the event had seen people being evacuated to hospital in a critical condition from heat stress and it seemed that it was one of those things that could never be predicted, as people react differently to the heat and humidity. With there being so many people in the event who spend all of their lives in cool dry climates, it was always a possibility that at least one of us would succumb to the tropical conditions.

As well as the race competitors and medical team

congregated in the Square, there were also several volunteer race support crew who would help out at checkpoints. The volunteer support crew don't get paid for their time spent helping out at the event. They even have to pay their own travel expenses. They all do it for the same reason as the competitors – to experience the mighty Amazon Jungle in a way the ordinary tourist never can. Some do it to see what conditions are really like so they can come back better prepared for when they run the event themselves. Whatever all the individual reasons people had for being there, everyone was on a level playing field now and we were all looking forward in eager anticipation to the adventure that lay ahead of us, once we boarded that river boat.

As it got later in the evening we all started to wonder exactly where we were meant to board the boat and if maybe it had arrived at a different part of the river and we weren't aware it was there. There didn't seem to be any organizers of the event in the Square and as time passed, groups of people started heading off down the street in the direction of the river in search of the boat.

While walking to the area we were told the boat would be leaving from, I ran into a group of Ice Marathoners who I had spent five days in Antarctica with the year before. Jason, Karen and Danielle were three of several competitors who were backing up the 2012 Antarctic Ice Marathon with the 2013 Jungle Marathon and like me, were now hooked on "destination" endurance events that not only take you to amazing locations around the world but also challenge you physically and mentally, taking you beyond your comfort zone and rewarding you with extraordinary experiences that redefine your boundaries on what's possible in life.

My Antarctic Ice Marathon friends were dining in a local street restaurant with a few more Jungle Marathoners and had just finished their meal, so we all started making our way down towards the riverbank to find the boat. I was relieved to see that some of these people probably had just as much luggage as myself, with one of them even carrying a large hard case containing a satellite phone and work gear at the request of their boss!

We walked to the end of the street and still couldn't see the boat or any of the other people who had walked down earlier, so we took a left turn back up to the main street before continuing down until we came to a communal area with a jetty, around which all the Jungle Marathoners were standing wondering when the boat would arrive.

A car full of young local people was parked along the side of the road amongst the crowd, with music blaring out of the windows as if providing entertainment for the hoard of backpacking visitors however, I'm sure many were thinking the same as me - that the music was deafeningly annoying and intruding on our conversations. Their revelry concluded with a comical moment though, when the locals went to start the car and found they had a flat battery from running the car stereo with the ignition turned off, so had to get a push start to go home!

The boat finally arrived, although I have no idea what time it came as I never looked at my watch. Knowing the exact time didn't seem to matter any more – it was either day time or night time – that was all you really needed to know.

The crowd was fairly quiet in the balmy tropical night air as we headed down the beach towards the dimly lit riverboat. It felt like a scene out of "The African Queen" as we approached the old timber boat called the "Natureza". A menacing toothy mouth was painted on the lower side of the bow as if to remind us we are entering piranha territory and leaving civilization behind for the next 9 days.

We boarded the boat in single file along a narrow wooden gangplank that stretched awkwardly from the lower deck of the boat to the sandy banks of the Tapajos River. The walkway was only about 18" wide, so it was quite a balancing act trying to carry all of my bags along the steeply sloping gangplank, all the while trying to hide the fact that my shoulders and back were caving under their weight and awkward size.

I was starting to feel a bit out of place amongst all of these seasoned adventurers, many of whom were extremely fit and camping-savvy ultra distance runners. I, on the other hand, am a self-confessed city-slicker who loves nothing more than a long indulgent hot shower before slipping into crisp hotel bed sheets after completing an exhausting marathon in a foreign city.

I knew this next week would be taking me further out of my comfort zone than I had ever dared to venture before. The thought excited me more than it scared me, although there were was a healthy dose of both emotions. Travelling on my own meant I had to pull my own weight, so I knew there was no point acting like a wimpy girl if the going got tough. No-one was going to help me string up my hammock, fight off the mosquitoes, carry me through the swamps or carry my pack – it was all up to me from here on, so I reminded myself of the saying "what doesn't kill you makes you stronger" and accepted my fate for the coming nine days as a Jungle Marathoner.

Once on board the boat it was a mad scramble to find a decent place to hang your hammock, with about 60 other people also trying to do the same thing. The old timber riverboat was constructed with large lower and middle levels and a smaller upper deck, with hooks positioned along the roof of each level for hanging hammocks.

The two top decks seemed to be already full by the time I arrived so I laid claim to two of the few remaining hooks near the aft of the lower deck. Unfortunately the bulk of the hanging hooks that remained were positioned adjacent to the engines, which were idling noisily beneath poorly soundproofed covers. Even more unfortunate for me though, was the exhaust outlet that funneled the diesel exhaust fumes from the engines below the bottom deck up into the crowded hammock-riddled first deck, right where the latecomers like myself had no choice but to settle in for the night.

I was secretly anxious about how successful I would be at this hammock-setting-up-and-sleeping thing as it was to be the first time I had ever done it. Sure, I got my newly purchased hammock out of the bag and took it to a local park a few days before leaving home, to make sure I knew how to tie it to a tree, but that 15 minute exercise was the limit of my experience. I was relieved that everyone was more preoccupied with trying to get their own gear organized than being conscious of my nervous attempt to look as if I knew what I was doing.

When I finally got the hammock strung up between two hooks, I took a deep breath before I awkwardly climbed inside it and gave it the first real test "run". I was relieved to find that the ropes didn't come undone and send me crashing embarrassingly onto the floor, like my doubting mind had convinced me was going to happen, and instead I hung there with the thin nylon fabric hugging around my body.

Due to the strong threat of malaria-carrying mosquitos, we were required to bring a hammock that had a fly screen attached to it, so the end effect was like being swathed in a nylon cocoon when you zipped yourself in. There were no home-style comforts like a pillow or sheets, just you and a piece of slippery nylon bending you into a banana shape while attempting to sleep. As it turned out, sleep was one thing I wasn't going to get that night!

Once I got my hammock hung and gear neatly stowed I started mingling amongst the crowd and sparked up a conversation with a couple whose hammocks were next to mine. Fred and Sandy were from Texas and Fred had attempted to do the Jungle Marathon the previous year but had been overcome with diarrhea and vomiting on the first day of the event and was unable to continue. He seemed unsure of what had caused it, but suspected it was from the poor sanitary conditions in the camps' ablutions area. This year he brought his wife with him and they were both going to attempt the 7-day event.

Setting up "camp" on the other side of my hammock was Mal, a true Jungle Marathon veteran who held the Veteran 60+ category record for the 7-day event.

Unfortunately though, he was only able to attend as a member of the support crew this year due to an operation on his hip earlier in the year. His advice left me more scared than better prepared, so I resigned myself to the fact that it was too late to act on any new information and I just had to accept my fate.

As the evening progressed with no movement of the boat, people started to question why the original departure time had been delayed. Word subsequently filtered through the crowd that we were waiting on a Japanese competitor who had gone fishing earlier in the day and had lost track of time after falling asleep, but he was now making his way to the boat.

People spilled out onto the beach, making conversation with new friends to kill the time. Moored alongside the 3-level "Natureza" was another smaller 2-level riverboat, which would be accommodating the race director and organizers, as well as the film crew from Rio de Janeiro.

The delay gave the cameramen a chance to test their drone camera, which was going to be used for taking overhead photos throughout the race. The contraption consisted of a framework of six arms, each with a helicopter-like propeller on top, and a camera suspended underneath. It was remotely controlled and the operator, who was standing on the top deck of the support boat, was maneuvering the drone above the water between the two riverboats. It's high-pitched motor attracted everyone's attention and people congregated along the port side railing of the boat to see what was making the noise.

You could barely make out the drone in the darkness

between the boats. If not for tiny lights on its edges it would have been invisible. It danced around above the water for several minutes until the operator must have been happy that it was a successful test flight, before he guided it down onto the deck in front of him.

The crowd went back to their subdued mingling and patiently waited for word that we would be heading off. It had been a very long day for most of the people as many had only flown into Santarem that morning or afternoon after a day or two travelling from various locations around the world.

I couldn't help but be reminded of a statement made in one of the newsletters we received in the months leading up to the event, where Shirley Thompson advised that once we get on the boat: "Relax, kick back and get into Brazil mode. Nothing happens at any great speed in the Amazon region, so switch off and enjoy being in such a picturesque part of the world". There was no doubt that timetables and schedules were not going to be a priority over the next nine days.

When the person we had been waiting for finally arrived, the gangplank was pulled onto the boat and it was time to start this adventure.

As I hung in the hammock I was trying to figure out if we had actually left the beach yet, because there was no feeling of the boat moving. After about an hour I realized that the suspended hammock was compensating for the movement of the boat, which meant no chance of motion sickness – yay!! I had finally found a positive in this otherwise sleepless and uncomfortable night.

We were told the boat would leave at about 11pm but

we never ended up getting away until after 1am. From then on, the days of the week disappeared from my mind and it didn't matter; we were in the Amazon Jungle with just one task ahead of us – to survive the next 9 days!

After travelling for about 5 hours upstream the boat headed for the sandy banks where we were to moor for a couple of hours to enjoy our first Amazon Jungle sunrise on the mighty Tapajos River. After dropping a metal ladder down the side of the boat, we all disembarked in the early morning twilight onto an amazing sandy beach where we stretched our legs and took in the wonderful dawn on the first day of our Amazon adventure.

The sandy banks showed signs of undisturbed wildlife that had been there before us, with a variety of footprints leading out from the foreshore bushes down towards the water. Discovering trails of jaguar footprints made me feel like an excited school kid exploring the world for the first time, snapping photos of my footprint next to the jaguars.

Some of the men came somersaulting off the top deck of the riverboat and splashed into the water next to the back of the boat, which acted as a signal to the rest of us that it was time for a dip, with many of us enjoying a relaxing swim in the fresh water shallows next to the boat. It was a beautiful warm morning and with the refreshingly tepid water being the closest thing we would have to a bath for the next week, I made the most of it.

I'm not sure if anyone else was thinking it, but I was hoping the boat would offer us some protection from any piranhas that might be lurking in the tropical Amazonian waters!

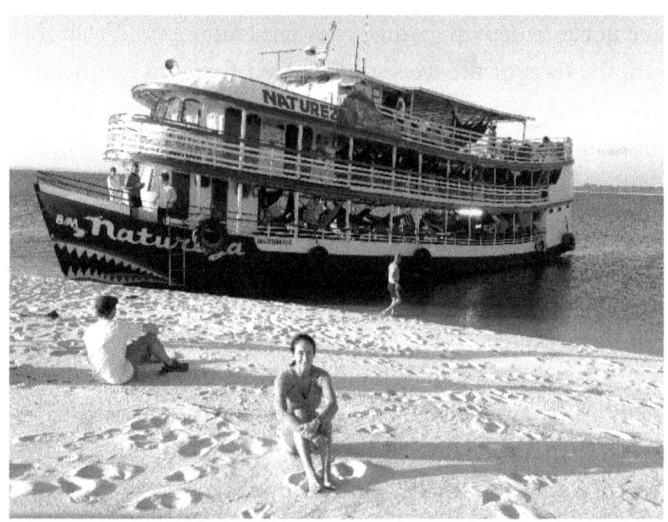

After about an hour on the sandbar, we all climbed back on board the boat and got comfortable for the remainder of the trip up the Tapajos River to our base camp, which would take another few hours.

Most of the hammocks had been taken down and packed away and people were chattier after mingling on the beach and getting to know the other competitors. Despite the fact that most people would have had very little sleep the night before, there was an air of excitement on the boat as the realization of the fact that we were finally in the Amazon Jungle took hold. The weather was perfect, with a beautiful breeze blowing through the open decks of the riverboat as the noisy, diesel-fumed engines powered us slowly along the river.

We had only travelled about a kilometer up the river when the boat started to turn around and head back to where we had just come from. It seemed we had left two people behind, who were around the back of the sandbar when the boat departed, and they didn't know we had gone. It was only through good fortune that there was another riverboat resting at the same location when we left.

The stranded Jungle Marathoners were able to get the people on that boat to radio our boat to let us know they had been left behind. Although it wasn't spoken out aloud, I'm sure many others were thinking the same as me, and wondering what would have happened if that other boat hadn't been there and when, or if, the two Jungle Marathoners would have been reported as missing. Upon thinking back to when we first left the beach, I couldn't remember our names being ticked off any list or a head count being done, although I'm sure the race director must have had some way of knowing who had boarded the boat at Alter do Chao and if any race participants were missing. With many of the participants travelling from around the world on their own, and the boat containing three levels of excited adventure travellers, it was easy to see how someone could have been missed.

It certainly served as a personal warning to make sure I didn't stray too far from the crowd in future and never assume someone was watching out for me. It's easy to get complacent when you are involved in an organized event, and just expect things to go smoothly without any involvement on your part, but this event clearly wasn't going to be any ordinary event.

There were to be no meals provided for the duration of the week in the jungle, so you were required to carry all of your own food. This meant that there were no designated meal times, although the race crew did boil water at various times for use in preparing the dehydrated meals that everyone had. The time on the boat was spent snacking on our camp food and brushing our teeth in the small communal basin on the bottom deck of the boat. It was time to get back to basics and enjoy the spectacular surroundings and the fun-spirited company of the fellow marathoners.

Prainha Base Camp – Day 1

After a few hours of slowly cruising along the Tapajos River, we started to make our way towards the shore at what was to be our base camp for the next two days and nights before starting the Jungle Marathon on the morning of the third day.

Children lined the banks of the river as the boat pulled to shore at the small community of Prainha. The Jungle Marathon supports a lot of the local villages that lie along the route of the event and the village people enjoy the attention they receive from the international adventure runners.

The children were all dressed in their very own Jungle Marathon t-shirts, and proudly lined up to welcome the guests as they carried all of their gear off the "Natureza" riverboat, made their way up the sandy banks of the river, along the tracks that wound around the small basic concrete shelters that housed the local people, and up to the campsite area about 200m into the jungle.

The village huts were very basic shelters constructed to mainly protect their food and scarce belongings from the weather, while most of their living and sleeping was done outside. Hammocks were strewn amongst the pole supports of the huts and under crude shelters that were erected to provide shade from the searing tropical sun. Despite the extreme heat and humidity the breeze did offer a pleasant relief if you were in a shady area, thanks to the cooling effect of your sweating skin.

An unfortunate side effect of colliding first world and third world cultures was the presence of packaged food wrappers strewn over the ground. It is a common sight in undeveloped cities, where processed and packaged food is such a treat, that they have no regard for the consequences of the litter when the packaging is discarded.

Thinking back to when I was a kid, it was also a common sight to see roadways strewn with rubbish in Australia. It escalated to the point where it was such a huge problem that an anti-litter movement took hold and littering became a fineable offense. Like most things I guess, there is a timeline that most trends follow and for these village people they don't yet appreciate the ugly side of packaged food.

When I first came across a wrapper on the path I picked it up out of habit and was somewhat ashamed to think that a visitor in my group had been so rude to throw away rubbish, but then I saw so much of it, and noticed most of it was old and weather-affected that I resisted the urge to pick up all the rubbish and just accepted it as a sad side affect of modernization.

With three large bags to carry, it was no easy task for me to negotiate the thick loose sand and rough dirt track up through the village, but I struggled on until I got to the campsite and then gladly dropped all my gear in a heap to let my overworked shoulders and back recover.

The campsite was a small cleared sandy area with dozens of tree trunks and additional poles set into the ground for use as hammock hanging points. These would be accommodating the 60+ hammocks belonging to the people who would be calling this patch of dirt home for the next 48 hours.

As was to become my arrival ritual at every campsite throughout the next week, the first thing to do was to find two trees from which to hang my hammock. With so many people vying for tree space it was sometimes difficult to find a suitable place. The campsites quickly became overcrowded with hammocks and the tie down ropes created quite an obstacle course.

As well as having a mosquito net on your hammock, you were also required to have a rain sheet which had to be tied over the top of the hammock with the ties either pegged into the ground or tied around suitable trees. These cords created a crisscrossing web of obstacles that Shelob or Aragog would have been proud of and which had to be either ducked under or stepped over as you walked around the campsite.

Once my hammock was hung up I placed my bags on the ground under it to try and keep them clear of the walkways, in addition to offering them some protection from the weather should it rain. The ground was covered in a sandy soil that was alive with tiny ants, and having open-toed shoes provided inviting flesh for the annoying ants to feast on. Their tiny stinging bites were more annoying than painful, so I decided to put my shoes and socks on to avoid the nips and any possible reaction or inflammation they might cause.

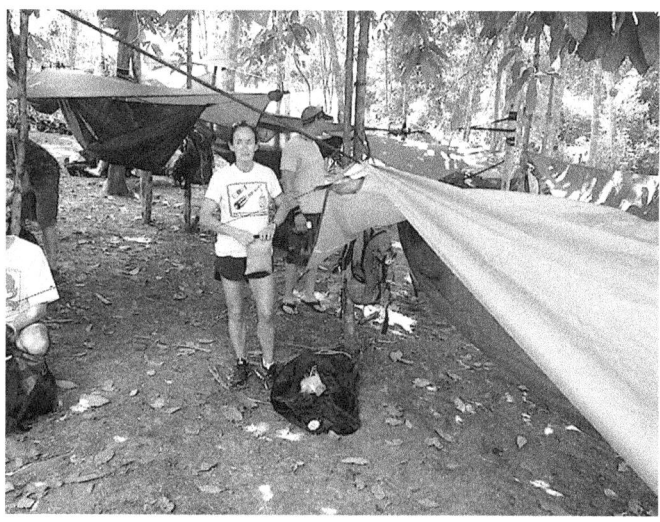

After spending several years working and living in tropical climates, I knew all too well how minor skin irritations could turn into serious infections. Invisible microscopic invaders can quickly become potentially life-threatening afflictions on unaccustomed immune systems. Even innocent scratches can become festering tropical ulcers in these conditions and over the next week our bodies were going to be pushed to physical exhaustion day after day, so any extra demands placed on our immune system could mean the difference between successfully completing the race or having to drop out.

The ants were not only on the ground but also crawling up the trees, so once my hammock was hung I sprayed insect repellent along all the cords connecting my hammock to the trees to try and stop anything crawling into bed with me. I also ensured the zip on my fly net was done up, whether I was in bed or not, to prevent any uninvited guests from joining me while I slept.

Now that I had my gear all organized it was time to explore the rest of the campsite. To the rear of the hammock area there was a thatched screen shielding the "long-drop" hole in the ground that would be our toilet for our stay here. With everyone having to use the one hole in the ground, it didn't take long for it to become a very unsavory place. There was no running water so you had to remember to take your wet wipes with you or else walk the 200m down to the riverbank to wash your hands afterwards.

The only permanent structure at the base camp was a shelter that was set up as a medic's station. The volunteer doctors had a large supply of first aid bandages and medications for everyday maladies, as well as intravenous equipment in the event of more serious life-threatening situations. Two ambulances were also on hand and would follow the Jungle Marathon route as closely as possible on the nearby road that runs parallel to the Tapajos River.

All runners were required to have a medical examination within 4 weeks of commencement of the Jungle Marathon, including an ECG test, the results of which had to be taken with you and checked by the medics before they would give the OK for you to start the event. The Amazon Jungle's heat, humidity and extreme terrain would prove to be unforgiving in the days to follow, so a clean bill of health was an absolute necessity before attempting to start an event that is arguably the world's toughest ultra-endurance race.

Once the medical paperwork was checked and all compulsory medical and gear checks were verified, you were given your two race number patches which had to be worn at all times throughout the race.

By the time I had completed all the organizational requirements it was mid afternoon and the tropical heat was starting to wear me down. I changed into my bikini and walked down through the village huts to the sandy banks of the river and into the shallows of the tepid, murky Amazonian tributary.

Although the Tapajos River is just a tributary of the Amazon River it is still an impressively wide waterway. It runs through the Amazon rainforest and, when combined with the Juruena River, the Tapajos is approximately 1,900 km long. The Tapajos River basin accounts for 6% of the water in the Amazon Basin. For its last 160 km it is between 6.4 and 14.5 km wide and much of it very deep. From where I was sitting it looked to be several kilometres wide, with the banks on the other side only barely visible.

There were already a few other Jungle Marathon people wallowing in the shallows, so I joined them. I went in deep enough to be able to duck my head under the water to cool off but didn't want to go any further out than thigh-deep, where I could just sit on the sandy bottom and relax. The fear of piranhas and other weird species of fish was fresh on my mind from watching TV documentaries on the Discovery channel, showing frenzied piranha attacks and mythical giant Amazonian fish that attack and kill small children who play in the murky-watered tributaries. Judging by the way no one else was venturing further out than thigh deep water I'm guessing they were all thinking the same thing. It seemed we were the brave few who even went that far, with the majority of the marathoners choosing to just put up with the heat and humidity rather than venture into the murky waters to cool off.

Although the banks of the river were very sandy, the surface below the water was slightly muddy and slimy so you had to walk around to try and find a patch that didn't feel too horrible under your feet. As the village we were staying at was quite primitive, I'm sure their effluent water would have been channeled into the river so it would be fair to say the river was not exactly a pristine waterway. There was also a lot of matter in suspension in the water so visibility was down to about 30cm. The thought of acquiring ear and eye infections from having your head submerged in the water kept me from doing it, except for rare brief dunking to cool off.

While cooling off I introduced myself to Mike and Marcus, two firemen from the UK, and Marieke from The Netherlands, who were also wallowing in the shallows. They were all volunteer support crew for the event and had paid for their own travel expenses just to be able to be a part of the Jungle Marathon adventure. Like the race competitors, the support crew also had to provide their own food and camp gear for the duration of the event.

The rest of the day was free time to get settled in the camp and relax. The cameramen once again trialed their drone camera and had it buzzing around above the campsite, getting a birds eye view of the tangled mass of hammocks and camp gear.

Some people chose to take advantage of a few showers that were set up down near the shore but as the water was most definitely being pumped from the river I couldn't see the point and I chose to just have another swim in the shallows of the river rather than having to line up and wait for a stand up version of the same.

I sorted through my dehydrated food packs to see what meal I had chosen for tonight's dinner and was concerned to find that after less than one day of eating these meals I was already baulking at them. The gourmet-sounding names on the packets made them out to be the camping equivalent of a Michelin-starred restaurant meal but to someone who only ever eats fresh food it was more akin to eating a bag full of rehydrated chemicals.

The fruit and porridge that I had for breakfast while on the riverboat was a sweet, gluey gunk and my evening casserole was a savory version of the same gunk. I can't believe I fell for the online marketing hype of the most expensive brand with the flashiest labels and overuse of the word "Gourmet". Then again, fresh food was out of the question so I didn't really have any choice.

I also had plenty of snacks but these tended to be mostly dried fruit, and after only one small pack of these the excessive sweetness was already getting to me. I started to wonder if I could possibly survive another 7 days on highly processed and sugary foods.

I couldn't help but think about how so many people in the world today live on similar highly processed and chemical-ridden packaged foods. From the snack food litter on the ground around the village huts that we were camped by, it was evident that the dietary scourge of the modern world had started to filter down to even remote parts of the Amazon Jungle. It would only be a matter of time before the addictive effects of trans fats and corn syrup, the stealthy toxic scourges of western world diets, would start to take it's hold on these peaceful, increasingly sedentary village people.

Before we all went to bed, the village children put on a cultural show for us down by the river and made the most of a rare opportunity to perform in front of an audience. Everybody was relaxed and enjoyed the jungle concert in the warm tropical surroundings of the Tapajos River. I could sense that everyone was quietly excited about spending their first night in the jungle, knowing that we still had another day to enjoy the scenery before the hard work began!

I was happy to have an early night after having next to no sleep the night before. After brushing my teeth in the bushes next to the hammock-hanging area, using my water bottle to rinse my mouth and spit into the bushes, I unzipped the fly net on my hammock and climbed in. The shorts and singlet I had been wearing all afternoon made do as pyjamas. I tried to take my shoes and socks off while hanging seated in the hammock in an attempt to avoid getting sand on my feet and subsequently in the hammock. This ritual would get discarded when racing through the jungle as I would be so exhausted at the end of the day that I wouldn't care less if there was a bit of sand sharing the hammock with me! At the beginning I held on to the little things that civilization makes you accustomed to – like no gritty stuff in the bed sheets.

When I laid down and zipped up the fly net it was quite warm in the hammock. I had no pillow or sleeping bag and just lay on the bare nylon fabric inside the zipped up cocoon.

The rain sheet was stretched out above the hammock and fastened to nearby trees in case it should rain overnight, but at the moment it was acting as a break from any tiny amount of air movement that might have otherwise given me some minor relief from the humid jungle air. I knew it would get cooler throughout the night and I thought I would most likely wake up shivering, so I kept a silk sleeping bag liner inside the hammock to slip into should this happen. Some hours later I was to find out that maneuvering into a slippery piece of silky fabric while bent into a banana shape and suspended between two trees is not an easy feat!

By early morning even the silk liner wasn't sufficient to keep me warm. The cooler morning air woke me up and had me trying to reposition the thin piece of slippery fabric around my shoulders while attempting to curl up into a fetal position and conserve body heat. I gave up trying to get comfortable – that just wasn't going to happen – but the intermittent sleep was still more than the "no sleep" I got the night before. I was not too concerned about the actual time spent sleeping and reassured myself that the total time spent laying in the hammock would provide enough rest and relaxation to counter any side effects of limited deep sleep.

At some stage during the early hours of the morning I awoke and after a few minutes I realized there was a weird sound in the distance. I lay there concentrating on the sound and tried to figure out what it was.

I had never heard anything like it before and the closest way I can describe it is that it sounded like a constant amplified, but distant, screaming noise or like the combined noise of thousands of screams way off in the distance. For what seemed like several minutes I strained my ears to try to figure out what the noise was but was at a total loss. Then I started to worry whether it was something that could be a threat.

The noise continued unabated and I convinced myself that if it was caused by something dangerous then surely someone would wake us all up and brief us on what to do. The longer it went on without any reaction from other people in the camp, the more I was able to relax, to the point I was even starting to think that maybe I was dreaming it – how could such a weird noise not stir everyone else up in the camp?? And then, without any cue, the noise abruptly stopped. There was dead silence, as if there was a tape recording of jungle noises being played at high volume off in the distance and had suddenly been turned off. I continued to lay there for some time, straining to hear if there were any other noises outside that might give me a clue as to what I had been listening to, but all that followed was silence and I eventually drifted back to sleep.

Prainha Base Camp – Day 2

As the advancing morning brought daylight into the green confines of my hammock, and the noise of fellow marathoners walking around close by became more prominent, I unzipped the fly net, swung my legs over the side and sat up on the edge of my hammock with my feet hanging down above the ant-riddled ground. I leant down to pull my socks on and after shaking out my shoes to ensure no creepy crawlies had sought refuge in them overnight, I lowered my feet into them and awkwardly stood up, clearing myself from the nylon web I had been hanging in.

Within a couple of hours of sunrise the early morning coolness gave way to the sultry tropical heat. With the race not starting until the next morning everyone was enjoying a relaxed start to the day and others emerged from their hammocks as their hunger, or bladder, dictated.

One of my closest hammock neighbors was Mel, the Jungle Marathon veteran, and as he had been here before I asked him if he heard the strange noise in the early hours of the morning and if he knew what it could have been. I was relieved to hear that other people had in fact heard it as well, so I wasn't imagining or dreaming it, and the consensus of opinion was that it was howler monkeys doing their thing.

Howler monkeys are native to South and Central America and are named, and known for, the loud guttural howls which they apparently use at the beginning and end of the day. They are considered to be the loudest animal in the world and while their howl isn't a piercing sound, it can travel for nearly 5km through dense forest. That would explain it! It seemed that my Google-searching son failed to pick up on that one – I guess it wasn't dangerous enough for him to be interested in.

There was very little to build a morning routine around in this no-frills accommodation, so once I emptied my bladder over the hole in the ground and brushed my teeth in the bushes, it was time to have some breakfast.

The race organizers had stocked the campsite with dozens of 20 litre water bottles to be used for cold drinking water and, after being boiled by the local women, hot water for dehydrated meals. A small table was set up next to the medic's shelter and people waited in line to be served what was to be our life blood for the next several days – clean water. Although we were required to bring iodine tablets for purifying drinking water if we ever needed to, there was more than enough bottled water to meet our needs at the campsites and the checkpoint stations throughout the days of racing. The iodine tablets would only be a back up if you were to get lost and needed to supplement your water from rivers or streams to get you by until you were reunited with the group. I was to find out in the coming days how real a possibility getting lost could be!

It was only the second morning of eating rehydrated breakfast meals and I was disturbed by how much I was not looking forward to eating another one. In fact, I didn't feel like any of the food I had and I knew the porridge and strawberries I had chosen was probably the best of a bad bunch. And as if the food's taste wasn't bad enough, it was pretty hard to judge exactly how much water to add to the foil pouches.

On the first day, I had left it up to the lady with the pouring jug and my ability to know when to say "woo", which was a big mistake. Practically all of my meals ended up being a watered-down sloppy mess and I'd be left using my fork to strain the chunky bits of food out of the watery mix. Some people were smart enough to use a measuring cup so they could add the exact amount of water the packet instructions recommended but I wasn't that well prepared. Instead, on day two I decided I would say "woo" a lot sooner and see how that would go. Although I managed to get a thicker consistency, I still found myself fighting the gag reflex from the taste and texture of the food. I was beginning to realize that self-supported multiday events probably weren't ever going to be my thing!

Once everyone was up and about and finished with breakfast, we all congregated in the village sheltered area for a briefing by the Chico Mendes Institute for Biodiversity Conservation (ICMBio). The ICMBio is a Brazilian federal government agency responsible for managing 313 federal conservation units and 15 research centres in Brazil. The ICMBio team gave a talk about the Institute, the National Forest of the Tapajos River and other protected areas in Brazil. This was followed by a lengthy presentation on the dangers we may be exposed to in the forest from both flora and fauna.

The elusive Jaguar would be a possible threat during Stage 3, as the race path and the deep jungle campsite we would be staying at that night encroached on their territory. For this reason there were to be armed guards maintaining a vigilant watch around the perimeter of the camp while the exhausted race competitors grabbed as much sleep as possible before the pre-dawn start to Stage 4.

There are also a variety of snakes that are prevalent in the rain forest and around the waterways, such as anacondas and the highly venomous coral snakes. Coral snakes are generally timid and will normally hear you coming and flee before you get a chance to see them but this may not always be the case, especially given that competitors will be running through forest tracks that are covered in leaf litter that could be refuge for a sleeping snake.

Trees and leaves are home for many insects and spiders whose bites can cause symptoms ranging from pain to serious or life-threatening illnesses. As previously described, the bullet ant is renowned as having the most painful bite of any known insect in the world, although it is not known to cause death.

There are also many spiders, which can be well camouflaged in the foliage and leaf litter, that can cause not only painful bites but, as in the case of the recluse spider, can also have serious necrotic flesh-eating effects, whereby flesh cells are killed and the body is unable to fight the affliction. The stomach-churning photos that were flashed up on the screen showing the effects of such necrosis hammered home the message about not sitting on the ground or holding onto trees or shrubs where these spiders might be hiding. Although we were unaware of it at the time, this message was to become even more pertinent to our group over the next 24 hours.

As if the fauna weren't dangerous enough, we also had to be very careful of many of the plants that we could be brushing up against while running along the narrow rainforest tracks. There were palm trees that had thorns more than an inch long lining their trunks and branches, and many other bushes also sported less-obvious smaller thorns. Even the leaves of the most common vines and shrubs were potential razor blades waiting to slice open the limbs of anyone who brushed along them in the wrong direction. These floral hazards reinforced the need to wear protective clothing on our arms, legs and hands to try and minimize the amount of damage that could be inflicted while traversing the unforgiving terrain.

With all of the race days having some sort of river, stream or swamp crossing, it was also important to know what threats were possibly lurking in the tributaries of the Amazon River. There was no surprise in hearing piranhas were in the waterways, as the souvenir shops in Alter do Chao had shelves full of stuffed and varnished piranhas for sale as a memento of your trip to the Amazon. I don't think there is anything more synonymous with the Amazon than the Piranha.

Caimans - Amazonian alligators – were also lurking in the waterways, and while they were good eating for the locals, we definitely didn't want to come across any while alone in the jungle. It was becoming clear why a part of the compulsory kit we had to carry with us was a sharp knife!

The film crew from the Brazilian adventure show were capturing every moment of the briefing on film as the large crowd of marathoners attentively listened to the talk, first in Portuguese, and then as it was translated into English. This was the first time we had actually been addressed as a group and it was exciting to feel a part of the epic adventure that was soon to begin.

A scan around the room showed mostly people between about 30 and 40 years old, which seemed to be typical for endurance events, and a handful of people who would have been over the 50-year old mark such as myself.

Nearly everyone was dressed in running shorts and

tank tops although many of the males were shirtless in the tropical heat. One standout competitor was a Japanese runner who was dressed from head to toe in a big furry black and white cow suit, complete with a fake cow head. Yoshi, as he came to be known, couldn't speak any English so no one was quite sure what the costume was all about. We couldn't help but wonder if he was actually going to run in the outfit, which seemed like an absolute impossibility given the extremely hot and humid conditions and that the course would have us crossing swamps and rivers. He sat through the presentation like a samurai warrior, without a hint of looking uncomfortable or a care about what anyone else may have thought about his inappropriate choice of jungle attire.

After the lectures were completed, it was time to get acquainted with the star of the show – a real live cobra. The presenter pulled over a box that had been sitting on the floor throughout the talk and carefully pulled out the agitated-looking snake for everybody to see. The Austrian competitor, Bernard, was chosen to "play" with the snake for the cameras and he was shown how to hold the reptile, with one hand firmly clamped just behind the head and the other supporting the rest of its body. Everyone, including the camera crew, swarmed in closer trying to get a good photo of the snake during the staged close encounter with an Amazon Jungle icon. If anyone was scared of the prospect of coming into contact with one of these beautiful creatures while running in the jungle it wasn't at all obvious – it was hard not to be fascinated by the remarkable creature.

With the jungle briefing out of the way, it was the

medics turn to brief us on how to survive the next seven days in the jungle environment. The heads of the medical team, Jeremy Joslin and Vicky Kypta, had lead the crew of medical volunteers at the Jungle Marathon for the past few years and knew exactly what the competitors were going to be up against.

We all knew the heat and humidity were going to be our biggest threats and the signs and symptoms of heat stress were explained to us so that we would hopefully know what to look out for. Signs of headache, nausea or disorientation were the alarm bells we had to watch out for and having adequate supplies of water and electrolytes would be critical in avoiding the threat. In past years competitors had been rushed to hospital in serious conditions from heat stroke and dehydration, so it was practically a given that there would be at least one person struck down at some stage given the lack of adequate acclimatization most people would have had. I'm sure most people were probably like me in thinking it wouldn't happen to them. Someone was going to be proven wrong in the next 24 hours!

Another cause for concern was what to do if you were unlucky enough to be bitten by a snake, especially if you were by yourself when it happened. With much of the route being inaccessible by vehicles it was important to keep moving and get to the next checkpoint as quickly as possible. All of the checkpoints were along roads that the ambulances could quickly access and then transport injured people to hospital in Santarem, if need be.

One other request was that we didn't consume any ibuprofen medication while running, although it was OK to use it once we were back at camp. Paracetamol was OK to take while running but the anti-inflammatory medications were not. Pain relief medication was likely to be a much needed commodity throughout the week ahead, and although all of the competitors were probably experienced endurance runners, many of them would not know how their bodies would cope with the added stress of the oppressive heat and humidity.

Without a doubt though, the most common complaint was going to be wear and tear on our feet and this year the medical crew included the services of ultra runner, and foot specialist, John Vonhof, the author of "Fixing Your Feet: Prevention and Treatments for Athletes". Blisters and lost toenails are a common occurrence in ultra distance events and the added complication of running in wet shoes and socks would only add to the discomfort. With river crossings, swamps and streams to be negotiated each day, there would never be a time when your feet would be dry so the likelihood of experiencing feet problems was extremely high.

Most of the presentations to the medic's tent at the end of each stage would be for foot related problems, so John was likely to be in high demand over the course of the next week. Preventative taping of hotspots on the feet is an important part of pre-race planning in ultra distance running and the competitors were advised to take all precautions necessary to avoid overwhelming the medics at the end of each day.

With the medic's talk competed it was time to collect our Velcro-strapped timing bracelets from the table and start preparing our gear for the race. We had until 5pm to sort out what we wouldn't need over the duration of the race and take this to the support boat for storage.

The way I tackled this was by laying out everything I had and once this was done I could see that I would need *three* 25-litre backpacks to carry it all, so the trick now was to decide which two thirds of the gear I would have to leave behind.

I started by gathering all the absolute essentials that we were required to take as per the rules because these were non-negotiable items. This included the compulsory medical and survival items, of which I had doubles of practically everything, so I rationed those out to the absolute minimum I thought I could get away with and placed them into a small dry sack to keep them safe through river crossings and in the event of rain.

The compulsory medical kit had to have Paracetamol, Imodium tablets, oral hydration salts, salt tablets, antiseptic cream, antiseptic wipes, sting/bite relief cream, plasters of various sizes, crepe bandage, 2 pairs of latex gloves, 5 x 20g needles and a pair of tweezers.

The rest of the compulsory kit items included a hammock with mosquito net and rainfly sheet, 2.5 litres of water carrying capacity, insect repellent, compass, safety pins, knife, torch and spare batteries, waterproof matches or lighter, water purifying tablets for at least 10 litres of water, emergency whistle and two cycalume glow/light sticks.

The essentials practically filled my 25-litre backpack, so I knew I was going to be struggling to fit everything in once I included food for seven days and personal items like clothes, toiletries and camera. Given that I was struggling to eat even one of the dehydrated food pouches each day, I was sure I wouldn't require the three I had originally allocated for each day, so I dropped it back to two a day as a compromise. Unfortunately these were packaged in foil sachets, which were quite heavy and bulky, but there seemed no way around this problem.

I also thought I would need a spare set of running clothes, a couple of T-shirts and a pair of shorts for in the camp in the evenings in addition to my bikini for swimming in the river. I didn't want to skimp on dry socks so I had packed a pair for each day. I also had a hat just in case we had any long stretches of the route out from under the jungle canopy and in direct sunlight. I don't normally wear a hat because it makes me feel too hot while running but I thought I could just hang it from the outside of my pack when I didn't need it.

There was no way all of this gear would fit in my backpack so I had to use all the outside pockets plus some small dry sacks that I clipped on the outside of my pack. I didn't think I could possibly cut back on any more gear than what I had so I was just going to have to live with this for the next week.

I packed up the rest of the stuff that I wouldn't need for the race and carried my big travel bags down to the boat for storage until I completed the event.

The rest of the day was spent mingling with the other competitors and relaxing in the shallow water along the riverbank. Considering the hot and humid conditions, I was surprised how few people were prepared to do the same. I could only guess that most people had concerns about piranhas and water-borne bacteria…. and probably rightly so!

By late in the afternoon I was anxious to get this day out of the way and start the race. As amazing as the Amazon Jungle was, being in a camp with no clean water for showers, no fresh food and no comfortable flat bed waiting for me at the end of another hot day wasn't my idea of a relaxing holiday. The first night in the hammock on the boat was the exciting start to this big adventure I had been planning for several months, the next night was like "Wow! I'm *really* sleeping in a hammock in the middle of the Amazon Jungle!!" but by the third night it was "I just want to get this race started!"

A meeting was scheduled for 5pm, to brief us on the course for Stage 1 so we would know what to expect the following day. The meeting point was down by the river, so everyone started congregating where we thought we were meant to be. However, it was some time before the race director, Shirley Thompson, finally appeared, slowly making her way along the sandy riverbank from the support boat and towards the group of waiting marathoners.

As she got closer we could see that she was being propped up on either side by a helper as if she was unable to support her own weight. When she finally stopped in front of us she stood on unsteady legs with a somewhat dazed look on her face. She apologized for being late and began to explain how a bullet ant had stung her earlier in the day, while doing a reconnaissance hike of the Stage 1 route we were to take the following day. While she was sitting on a log for a rest she said she had felt something sting her through her pants and when she looked to see what it was she found a large ant that she would later learn was a "bullet" ant – named on account of its powerful and potent sting.

The locals call it the "Tucandera" or "24 hour ant", referring to the 24 hours of pain that follows being stung. The ants are generally between 18-30 mm long and resemble stout, reddish-black wingless wasps. The effects of the sting have been described as "waves of burning, throbbing, all-consuming pain that continues unabated for up to 24 hours". The venom of the bullet ant contains a paralyzing neurotoxic peptide, which affects voltage-dependent sodium ion channels and blocks the synaptic transmission in the central nervous system.

As the pain migrated from the sting site to all around her body, Shirley knew this was much more than an ordinary old ant bite. The medical team met her with the ambulance and hooked her up to intravenous pain relief but she said this barely took the edge off the intense pain. It took a few hours for the neurotoxic effects of the venom to wear off to a dull bearable level of discomfort, even under the influence of the heavy duty painkillers she continued to be drip fed.

Shirley later described the pain as being like a continuous electric shock pulsating through her body, which was agonizingly debilitating in its intensity. Unbeknown to the competitors, Shirley spent all afternoon hooked up to a morphine drip in the ambulance and our race briefing was the first time she had been up and about since the incident.

The race director's unfortunate encounter with the local wildlife was a timely reminder to us all about how dangerous the harsh environment could be. I couldn't help but smile at the thought of how excited my son would be when he heard that a bullet ant had bitten someone, although I knew Shirley would have been much less excited about having just "taken one for the team"!

Shirley briefed us on logistical aspects of the race and explained how the course would be marked with flagging tape which would be visible at all times, such that if we could not see any markers then it was important to stop and retrace our steps back to where we saw the last piece of marker tape before trying again to find the next piece. While this sounded very reassuring, my hopeless sense of direction meant that I was to learn in the days to follow that finding these pieces of marker tape could prove harder than it was made out to be.

The race rules were explained and everyone was reminded that the Jungle Marathon is a fully self-supported race. We were advised later in the afternoon we were going to have to load any gear that we wouldn't need for the duration of the race onto the support boat, where it would stay until the race was finished. Everything you kept after that had to be carried in your backpack for the duration of the race – food, medical kit, clothes, hammock, rain sheet, and any personal items. The more you kept, the more weight you had to carry around in your backpack everyday.

We also had to have 2.5 litres of water carrying containers on our bodies at all times and that these were to be full at the start of each stage and be topped up at checkpoints. Dehydration and heat stress were real dangers in this environment and it was critical that we carried enough water to get us to each checkpoint.

Our gear would get checked at the start of each stage to make sure we were starting with 2.5 litres of water each day. The organizers were concerned that people would skimp on water to decrease the amount of weight they had to carry while racing and then face the risk of running out before getting to the aid stations.

A first for this years' event was the addition of timing wristbands that would also double as checking devices to try and stop people from cheating and taking shortcuts through the jungle that they weren't meant to take. It was a well-known fact that in previous years some of the local Brazilian competitors would cheat by taking shortcuts, meeting up with people in the jungle who would carry their gear for them or even hitch a lift on motorbikes.

It was hard to believe that anyone would go to such lengths to cheat at this type of event and I'm sure all the "foreign" competitors were like me, taking on endurance events as a personal challenge to push yourself to see what you're physically capable of. The other competitors are what make you dig deep and not give in. Cheating to pass them would be such a hollow victory. However, obviously not everyone thinks like this and there was a cultural divide that threatened the fair and honest runners from possibly achieving the hard earned results they deserved.

To try and combat this problem there were to be secret checkpoints along the course that required swiping your timer as proof that you had followed the flagged track, but it still wasn't a foolproof way of completely eliminating the chance of someone cheating elsewhere in the jungle. Short of wirelessly tracking every competitor, it was always going to remain a problem when some of the competitors were locals who would be running on their home turf and would know the tracks in the forest like the back of their hand – a fact I would personally find out the next day when we started stage one. The message was well and truly spelt out to all the competitors that cheating would not be tolerated and would result in either a disqualification or time penalties.

Shirley briefed us, first in English and then in Portuguese for the benefit of the many Brazilians who didn't speak English, on what we'd be up against in Stage 1, and explaining the terrain conditions between each of the four checkpoints.

Although the first stage was only 23km, it would be a short sharp shock to the system, giving us a taste of everything the jungle can throw at us. It would include water crossings, steep hills, swamps, jungle trails and would pass through one of only three indigenous communities in the Tapajos National Forest, known by the locals as the FLONA (Floresta Nacional do Tapajos).

As a precaution to prevent people from overdoing it on the first day and risking heat stress, it was compulsory for all competitors to rest for 15 minutes at each checkpoint before continuing on. This time would be deducted off our final time at the end of the day. It was again stressed that any cheating would result in disqualification and that there was a secret checkpoint that everyone had to pass through as proof that they were following the correct route.

With the race briefing out of the way and all of our extra gear packed away on the boat, the atmosphere had shifted from laid back camping mode to "nervous energy" mode as the start of the 2013 Jungle Marathon drew closer. Even though the Jungle Marathon is a competition and one that the most experienced athletes take very seriously, the solidarity amongst the competitors was strong as people shared equipment tips and strategies on how to better survive the race.

It was easy to pick the experienced multi-day ultra runners, as they had the most compact backpacks with the least amount of gear. These guys knew exactly what they would need and wouldn't be burdened with the "just in case" items that first-timers like me would be packing. To say I was starting to feel "out of my depth" would be an understatement but I also knew that the bigger the challenge, the greater the reward. I just wanted this challenge to start – the hanging around waiting for it was getting to me.

With the morning's final race preparations having to begin in the pre-dawn darkness, it was essential to have all of your race gear fully prepared before going to bed. We were stripped down to the bare essentials so that wasn't going to be too much of a drama, although some people could be heard stressing over how to fit everything into their backpack and how heavy it was. I was glad I wasn't the only one!

By early evening I was eager to get to bed and try to fast-forward the next 12 hours so we could finally get started on this race. The longer I lounged around thinking about it, the more worried I got about possibly not being prepared enough for the event. Any extra time spent "roughing it" in the jungle before the race was just going to wear me down physically and mentally from lack of fresh food and a comfortable bed.

It had also been several days now since I had done any

running, due to all the travel, so I was starting to feel lethargic and badly wanted to get moving. The lack of daily routine and wholesome nutrition was starting to feel like as big a challenge as the race itself for me and, as much as I wanted to embrace the whole camping-out-in-the-jungle experience, I had to admit that I would enjoy the Amazon a whole lot more from a five star riverboat cruise. My mind was already starting to mess with my head and the race hadn't even started yet!

Chapter 5

RACE DAY – STAGE 1

Prainha to Pini – Approximately 23km

Stage 1 Brief

Start (Prainha) to Checkpoint 1 (Igarape): 4.97km
Checkpoint1 to Checkpoint2 (Casa Heraldo): 2.61km
Checkpoint 2 to Checkpoint 3 (Takuara): 5.16km
Checkpoint 3 to Checkpoint 4 (Fazenda): 3.46km
Checkpoint 4 to Finish (Pini): 6.57km

There will be a compulsory 15 minute break at each checkpoint

---

After waking several times during the night and checking my watch to see what the time was, I finally heard other people moving around at about 5am so I disentangled myself from the silk sleeping bag liner, washed down the daily dose of anti-malarial drug, and unzipped my hammock before standing up to greet the first day of the Jungle Marathon.

With the race not starting until 7am I still had plenty of time to have breakfast and change out of my sleeping clothes and into my race clothes. After visiting the hole in the ground for my morning relief, I took a pouch of

RACE DAY – STAGE 1

dehydrated porridge up to the water table to let the boiling water work it's magic. I knew I had to try and eat as much as possible before starting the race so I force-fed myself the gooey gunk in the pouch until I couldn't stomach it any more.

With the help of a headlamp I started organizing my race clothes in the predawn darkness. Changing from my sleeping clothes into my racing clothes was done standing next to my hammock and I just hoped that everyone was too busy organizing themselves to pay too much attention to a lady stripping off amongst them.

I wore a lycra tank top that covered my abdomen and a pair of nylon/lycra calf length tights. To protect the lower part of my legs I wore knee high compression socks that had a stirrup foot on them. Once these were on, I put my Saucony trail runners on and then a pair of lycra gaiters over the top of my shoes to prevent dirt or creepy crawlies from falling into my shoes. Just before we started the race I planned on donning a long-sleeved lycra front-zipping jacket to protect my arms from scratches, stings and sunburn, and then a pair of fingerless training gloves to protect my hands. Although it was going to be very hot and humid, I didn't want to have any of my skin unprotected from all the hazards and dangers we were likely to be exposed to in the jungle. I layered my clothing such that if I got too hot then I could easily peel off layers as need be. Everything was made of nylon or lycra in an effort to avoid being weighed down by wet clothes after river and swamp crossings, as well as from the sweat we would be covered in.

Once my clothes were all organized it was time to pack up my hammock and rain sheet. I still wasn't sure how much room these would take up in my backpack so had to make sure I wrapped them up as tightly and compactly as possible. I filled up my 2-litre water bladder and placed that in the backpack first, with the opening side facing up so it could be refilled at checkpoints without having to pull everything out of the pack to access it. The hammock then went in, followed by the medical kit, food and the few clothes I was taking. There was no way I could fit everything inside the pack so I had to hang some of the dry sacks on the outside. I used all the outer pockets to store things like my camera and snacks to eat while I was running. Once everything was packed, I grabbed the top of the pack and lifted it up off the ground to test how heavy it was. I guessed it to weigh about 13-14kg, which is about 30% of my body weight, so it was not going to be fun lugging this around on my back all day. The only training I had done with a backpack was with a weight of about 4kg so I knew this would be a big handicap. I was here though, so there was nothing else to do but get on with it.

Using the safety pins that were part of the compulsory kit we had to take with us, I pinned one of my race numbers to the outside of my backpack so it was visible from behind and pinned the other to the top of my leggings so it would be out of the way of my pack straps. It was compulsory to have both race numbers clearly visible at all times throughout the event.

The start line was on the riverbank so I made my way down the rough dirt pathway that wound through the village huts. As I walked past one of the medics she commented on how heavy my backpack looked and grabbed it to feel for herself. "*You can't run with that!*" she yelled at me in disbelief, "*It must weigh nearly as much as you do*." She seemed so surprised by the weight of my pack that for a moment I thought she was going to intervene and say I couldn't start the race. I just shrugged and said there was no way I could make it any lighter and continued walking.

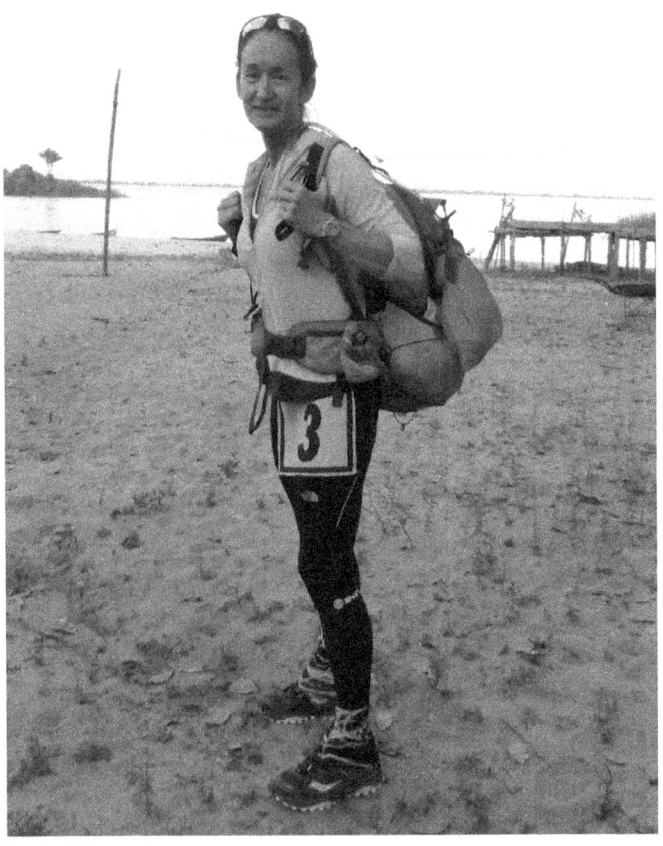

Once I got down to the starting area my backpack was checked by one of the race volunteers to make sure I had the compulsory 2.5 litres of water and medical supplies, although it was nearly impossible to tell for sure because everything inside was well packed.

Along with the 2-litre water bladder inside my pack, I also carried a 500ml water bottle that I stored in one of the outside pockets. I had so much gear jammed into the pack I was worried that the zip would pull apart against the strain of it all.

Up until now I hadn't tested the weight of the pack on my back because I didn't want to have to carry it any longer than I really needed to but now it was time to strap it on and accept my fate. Getting it up was probably the hardest part however, once it was on and the straps were tightened as much as they could be, it didn't feel too bad. The fully tightened straps made the pack sit up high on my back and it actually felt quite comfortable.

With all the gear checks done it was time to assemble behind the "START" banner, which was propped up on poles in the sand. There were 59 people starting today with 16 of those (10 males, 6 females) competing in the 4-day 120km event and 43 (38 males, 5 females) doing the full 7-day 250km event. Those only doing the stand-alone 42km (marathon distance) event on day 4 would join us on the day. The drone camera was buzzing overhead filming the excited competitors assembling into place. Finally, after the race director wished us all good luck, the countdown was completed and the horn sounded for the start of the 2013 Jungle Marathon.

RACE DAY – STAGE 1

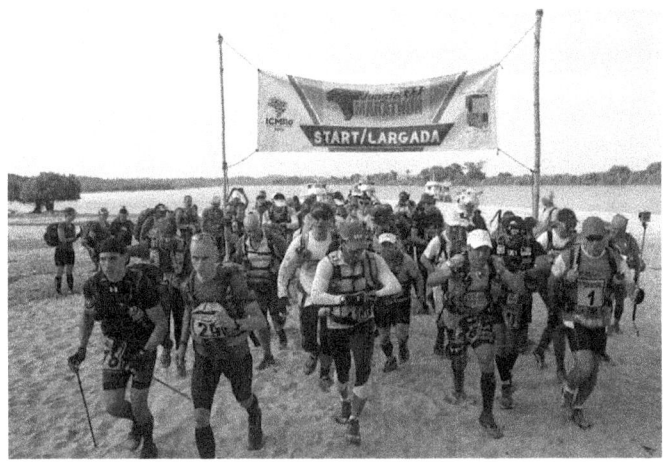

I jogged at the rear of the group as we wound our way back up the path through the village and around the area we had been camping in, before starting a gradual climb up into the jungle. The track wasn't very wide so it wasn't long before everyone was in single file and had settled into a comfortable pace. The track was well worn but there were many tripping hazards to watch out for, like exposed roots, rocks and washouts. The first day's stage was meant to be only 23km but given the extreme terrain we were expecting to pass through, it was impossible to estimate how long it would take to complete.

After running for only a few minutes I caught up to Carol, the journalist from the Planeta Extremo filming group, who had been stopped by a young boy who asked if he could have his photo taken with her. Apparently the show is quite popular in Brazil and it would not surprise me to learn that the young and beautiful star of the show is quite a celebrity in her native Brazil. It was hard to imagine that the village we had just left even had a television, so I'm not sure where the boy was from and how he could have known who she was. After a quick photo with the young fan she was back running with her Planeta Extremo co-star, Clayton.

The 5km leg to checkpoint 1 was on gently undulating jungle tracks that were clearly flagged with tape. I hadn't paid any attention to the tape at the start because I was busy watching my feet so I didn't trip over the many trip hazards along the path, and as I was in the rear of the pack I just followed the people in front of me, trusting that they were all heading in the right direction.

A couple of kilometres into the race, I automatically followed the two runners directly in front of me as they ducked under a strip of blue flagging tape that stretched across the track leading off to the left. I thought it was strange that the race organizers would flag the track in this way and have us ducking under the tape but my brain must have already decided it was better to keep following the people in front of me rather than trust my intuition.

After another few minutes another runner ran past me, and as he did, the man I was following stopped and looked around and commented on not having seen any tape markers for a while. The three of us stopped and called out to the man who was up ahead of us that we had no tape along the track and we may have taken a wrong turn. The man who was directly in front of me commented that it must have been where that blue tape was stretched across the track, so we turned around to back track. The man out ahead who we had all been following was calling back in Portuguese and the other Brazilian who was with us yelled out that we were going the wrong way. They conversed for a few moments in Portuguese as two of us headed back the way we had come. I turned around to see both of them continue on the way they were going so it suddenly dawned on me that the Brazilian guy who was leading us down the wrong track must have known all along he was off the marked track and he was taking a shortcut. I couldn't see any other explanation for why he would keep going when it was clear we were on the wrong track. Anyone who wasn't familiar with the terrain wouldn't dare to take an unmarked track in the Amazon Jungle unless they knew where it headed, so a cheating competitor seemed like the only possible explanation for the strange behavior.

I picked up my pace to match that of the UK competitor who had been in front of me while following the Brazilian, as we ran back to where the blue tape was over the track. We were annoyed with ourselves for not using our common sense when we ducked under this obvious barricade the first time we encountered it. We were even more annoyed at the fact that someone else's possible cheating had made us lose time in the race.

After briefly introducing ourselves to each other, I continued to jog behind Alfredo as we overtook a few people in an effort to make up a bit of the time we had lost. The track was really only wide enough for single file so if you wanted to pass somebody you had to excuse yourself so they could move into the bushes to let you pass. Despite the weight of my backpack I was surprised that I was able to maintain a steady jogging pace. I decided to try and stay with Alfredo for as long as I could so I had someone to pace me and keep me from slacking off to a walk.

After running for several minutes I noticed one of my waterproof pouches drop on the ground next to me, so I picked it up and strung the cord around my neck for now. It contained my Malaria medication and my toothpaste and toothbrush. I couldn't remember which pouch I had shoved it into so I thought I'd just wait until I got to the first checkpoint and use the compulsory 15 minutes break to sort it out.

Within a few steps, I noticed that my pack felt a bit weird, as if it was lopsided or something. Just as I was making sense of the shifting weight on my back I heard calls from people behind me telling me what my mind had just figured out – my pack had come undone and everything was falling out of it while I was running! As I let out an exasperated yell, Alfredo stopped to see what was wrong but as I knew this was going to take some time to fix I told him to keep going and not wait for me.

My worst fear when I saw the gaping opening was that the zip had pulled apart because my backpack had been so tightly packed. If this had happened then I would not be able to carry all of my gear and the race would have been over for me, so for a few moments an overwhelming sense of despair raced through my body. Further inspection revealed that the zip had just come undone and relief replaced the despair. I quickly shoved all the contents back inside the pack so I could continue to the checkpoint.

It wasn't long before I reached checkpoint 1, which was next to a beautiful swiftly flowing stream of clear water. We were deep in the jungle and the humid air was very still under the dense canopy. My name was ticked off a checklist and the arrival time noted so they could let me know when my 15 minutes of rest was up and I could be on my way.

The race volunteer manning this checkpoint was a British guy who was smoking a cigarette while keeping tabs on everyone. It was impossible to avoid breathing the cloud of smoke he produced that permeated the still and moisture-laden air in the small waiting area, which was bounded by dense, low-lying vegetation and the sandy riverbank. I had no choice but to suck it up as I needed to focus on organizing my pack so it sat comfortably on my back again.

I realized that my mistake had been to zip my pack with both zips meeting at the top, making it very vulnerable to bursting open. Certainly a rooky mistake, which seemed so obvious in hindsight that I was embarrassed even thinking about how stupid a mistake it was. Once everything was packed back in as neatly as possible, I zipped it up and made sure both zips were together at the bottom of one side. Alfredo, who was still waiting for his 15 minutes of rest time to pass, gave me a small cable tie to thread through the two zips so they would not come apart again. It seemed Alfredo was like a modern day MacGyver and he had a little bag of bits and pieces to get him through any gear malfunction. I was very grateful for his help.

While I was fixing my pack, the two Brazilians whom we had followed down the wrong track earlier, walked into the checkpoint, so their shortcut didn't seem to have given them any advantage. I wanted to give them the benefit of the doubt but it just seemed too unlikely that the man in front would have kept going when it was obvious we had strayed from the correct route. Maybe they did in fact eventually backtrack and resume the correct path but I wasn't going to confront them and ask if they cheated, even if I could speak Portuguese.

After my 15 minutes was up, my name was called and it was time to continue the race. We had to cross the stream in front of us and there was a rope strung across it to help us negotiate the swiftly flowing water. It was hard to tell how deep the water was but if it was deeper than waist height then I wanted to put my backpack in a dry sack so I could keep the water out of it.

I asked the man at the checkpoint how deep it was and he indicated it was only up to about waist height however, my waist is a lot lower to the ground than most other people's. I was sure it wouldn't take much to lose my balance in the current or trip on submerged rocks or logs, which would have meant my pack going under water for sure.

I decided to take the time to stuff it into a large dry sack I had in one of the outside pockets. I scrambled down the bank and into the stream, which was only about 10-15m wide, but as I suspected the bottom was very uneven and in one step I went from waist deep water to being unable to feel the bottom. I only stayed afloat thanks to the buoyancy of my air-filled dry sack.

The water was surprisingly cold and took my breath away when I suddenly found it up around my chest. There were two cameramen on the other side of the stream filming and photographing everyone as they came across, no doubt getting some great shots as unwary people sank under water when the stony bottom disappeared from beneath their feet.

As soon as we emerged from the stream we stepped straight into a swamp that extended into the darkness of the jungle ahead. It was impossible to carry my pack while it was inside the dry sack so I took it out and reset it on my back, freeing up my hands to help steady me as I negotiated the swamp.

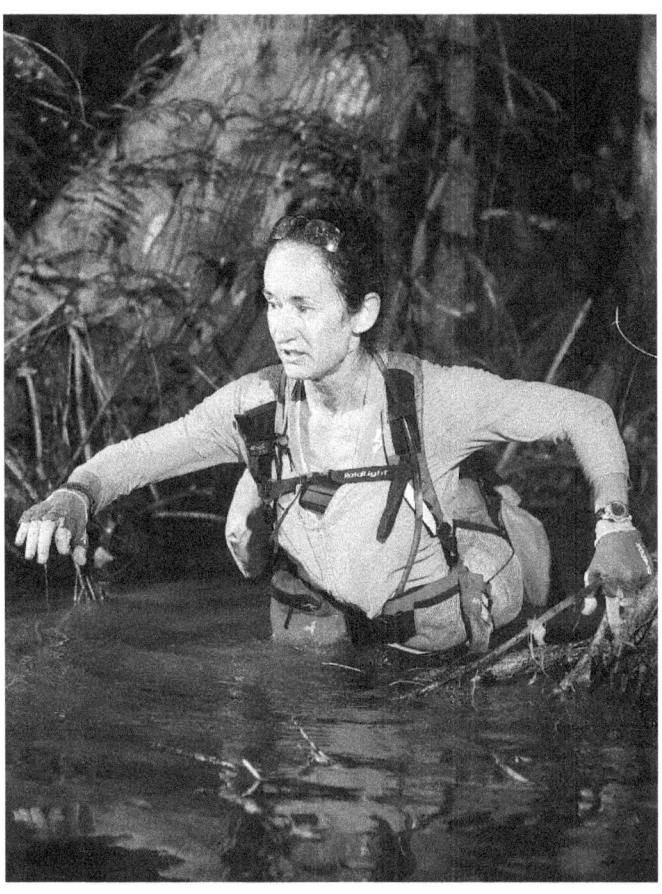

A muddy pit full of roots and logs stretched out in front of me and on the opposite side of it was another group of cameramen. I had no idea if I was supposed to try walking through the swamp or go around it. I stood stunned for a minute while I figured out how I was meant to get to the other side. It seemed incomprehensible that I would have to venture into the unknown depths of the swamp, not being able to tell how deep it was and there being nothing to hold on to if I was to lose my balance and fall over. The cameramen were cheering me on and I felt like I was in a reality TV show only it was shockingly all too real! I knew I had no choice but to toughen up and just do it.

Despite knowing that we would be having to negotiate Jungle Amazon swamps leading up to the event, nothing can prepare you for how you feel when you actually have to do it. If it weren't for the cameramen's floodlights, the area would have been extremely dark. This was very dense jungle terrain with correspondingly abundant jungle wildlife – nothing nice could possibly live in this inhospitable environment. The thought of being waist deep in slimy mud in the Amazon Jungle was like my worst nightmare becoming reality – but now I had to live it. I trudged through a waist deep cesspool of mud, animal faeces and rotting vegetation, not knowing with each step if the firm ground underneath my feet would suddenly disappear and send me sinking in over my head.

I was terrified of getting one of my shoes stuck in the deep mud and having it pulled off my foot because I was sure I would never be able to retrieve it. I had done my shoelaces up extra tight before starting, just to minimize the risk of this happening, but the suction forces in this formidable liquid could not be underestimated. I was grateful for the long sleeves and total leg coverings and hoped these would prevent any insidious little swamp critters from taking a liking to any bare flesh. Keeping all orifices and crevasses covered by a layer of lycra was essential to prevent things from crawling into places they had no right to be. Every step was an effort, both mentally and physically, as I struggled to maintain my balance and keep moving against the resistance of the thick mud.

Finally we left the swamps behind and continued along the dark jungle track. I had been on my own since crossing the stream and remained this way until arriving at checkpoint 2, which was a distance of only 2.6km but over extremely challenging terrain.

There was another compulsory 15-minute rest stop here so I topped up my water bottle and took my pack off my back and lay down on the ground to rest. My back was starting to ache from the weight of my pack and lying down was welcomed relief for my back and legs. The heat and humidity crept up as the morning progressed but fortunately the dense jungle canopy kept the hot sun off us most of the time. It was only when I emerged out of the trees and crossed over the dirt road to get to the checkpoint, that I noticed how hot the morning had become. Despite all the layers of tight clothing I was wearing, I wasn't too bothered by the heat and humidity and hoped this would continue. I was prepared to take my long sleeved lycra top off if necessary, but only as a last resort if I thought I was over-heating. Having a layer of fabric between my skin and the jungle flora and fauna seemed a higher priority at that stage, as I knew even the slightest flesh wound could deteriorate with severe consequences in this environment.

Once my name was called I headed off back into the jungle for the 5km hike to checkpoint 3. The jungle terrain was starting to take it's toll on my legs and having to watch every step I took to prevent tripping over numerous stumps and vines made the job of watching out for flagging tape in the trees all the more difficult.

Despite being told at the pre-race briefing that we would be able to see the next piece of tape from an adjacent one, this was sometimes not the case. Most of them were very small and looked like they had been in the jungle from previous year's events because they were faded and blended in with the jungle colors so well. With the field of competitors spaced out considerably already, I found myself alone with no one else visible in front or behind me, so I had to be really careful not to take a wrong turn.

By the time I got to checkpoint 3, my back and neck were really aching and all I wanted to do was remove the burden on my back and lay down. I dropped down onto a blue tarpaulin that was spread out under the shade of some trees and tried to relax but all I could think about was having to put that pack back on in 15 minutes. Even lying flat didn't provide much relief and muscle spasms were distracting my mind from everything else that was going on around me. I drank from my water bottle and had a bit of a snack, trying to distract my mind from the pain, but all I could think of was how hard it was going to be just to finish today's stage, let alone another 5 stages over the next

RACE DAY – STAGE 1

6 days!

As I looked around at the other competitors taking a break at the checkpoint, I couldn't help but notice that one of the men had an extremely red and flushed face. Although my back and legs were trashed, the heat still hadn't really bothered me and no one else seemed to be red-faced either. As well as looking very hot, the man seemed to have a slightly disoriented look about him, which struck me as being a possible sign his body was struggling to cope with the heat and humidity.

Although the medics would be looking out for signs of distress that could indicate a runner may be facing problems, they knew that ultra distance runners are not the type of people to give up at the first sign of pain or discomfort. Their job was to do everything they could to help the competitors achieve their goal of completing the Jungle Marathon. They were well aware that at any time they could be faced with a situation where they have to make a judgment call on whether a person could safely carry on or risk possible life-threatening consequences if they attempted to. Physical injuries, like snake bites or heavy bleeding, can make this decision a no-brainer but the subtle changes that heat stress can have on your body are impossible to definitively evaluate as every person reacts differently.

Like altitude sickness, it's impossible to predict who will be affected by it so the medics had to keep a close watch for telltale signs that the runners themselves may not even notice. With all the checkpoints being manned by a few medics and also a few non-medical volunteers there was a big emphasis on using your 15 minutes of compulsory rest time to re-hydrate and cool down as much as possible. People were there to help fill your water bottles and were even offering to pour a jug of water over your head if you felt it would help. Heat stress can turn into heat stroke very quickly and if this deterioration occurs, then you need to get to hospital urgently. The harsh jungle conditions made it a near certainty that everyone would be affected by heat stress to a certain degree but the medics couldn't just pull people out of the race because they had a red face. The line between heat stress and heat stroke is a very hazy one and it was probably safe to say that no one would stop a competitor from continuing unless they were so badly affected they couldn't speak for themselves. Needless to say, everyone continued through checkpoint 3.

The 3.5km between checkpoints 3 and 4 continued along dense jungle tracks, with some sections flat or undulating whereas other sections were ruthlessly steep. For a region that has no mountains, it was surprising how hilly the route was in places, and the hill sections were mercilessly unforgiving on my legs and back. The near-vertical climbs were on leaf-littered tracks that provided little traction for your feet. You had to try and place your feet where other runners had already stepped, creating small patches of dirt that the ball of your foot could use to push off against.

Small trees along the side of the track provided anchor points to help pull yourself up but you had to try and watch out for thorns or biting insects. I was hoping my fingerless gloves would provide enough protection should I clamp down on something without realizing it. The bigger trees offered a chance to have a brief break by leaning against them, which stopped you from tumbling back down the hill. The steepness all but prevented you from being able to halt part-way through a climb without having something to hold onto.

While struggling to make it up one of the climbs, I was surprised to see the Russian competitor, Anna, coming down the hill towards me. She had no pack on and when I asked what she was doing she said there was an injured runner up ahead and that she was going back to checkpoint 3 to alert the medics. All I could think of was how spritely she looked and that she would have to repeat this climb to finish stage one. I couldn't help thinking that I would never have been able to do that and what an amazing good Samaritan Anna was.

My body was under such duress while climbing the seemingly never-ending hill that I had gone past the injured runner without even realizing it. He was sitting on a big fallen tree that crossed the track and the Brazilian journalist, Clayton, was waiting with him. Carol, the journalist who was running with Clayton, had continued ahead to alert the medics at checkpoint 4. The injured Venezuelan runner, Pedro, eventually got to checkpoint 4 where one of the lead medics, Jeremy, cleaned and stapled the wound such he was able to continue running, despite the injury.

Finally I came out of the jungle and the marker tape led down a dirt road, which was exposed to the hot midday sun. The flat sandy surface of the road was a welcome relief after the steep hills and slippery surfaces under the jungle canopy. My back and shoulders were screaming in pain and my legs were getting very tired as well due to the extreme terrain and the unaccustomed burden of the extra 15kg of baggage weight.

I wanted to take advantage of the nice flat road and break into a jog but there was no way I could find the strength to do anything except place one foot in front of the other and be happy that I was still moving forward. I had a small boost to my spirits when I could see Checkpoint 4 up ahead and, upon entering the rest area on the side of the dirt road, I managed to give a forced smile to the volunteers and medics as they called out my name and ticked it on their list.

I went straight to the blue tarpaulin that was stretched out over the embankment and released my backpack so I could sit down and get the weight off my back and legs. I sat uncomfortably against the mound of dirt and sucked on some warm water as a sign to the medics that I was still functioning OK. I was sure nothing could have masked the pain I was feeling though. Knowing that a 15 minute rest would barely make any difference to my aches and pains made it even harder to pretend I was happy.

There were no other runners waiting at the roadside stop as the competitors were well spread out by this time of the day. Many of the faster ones would already have finished and be at the camp site setting up their hammock and recovering, while I was contemplating the torture I still had to go through before I could enjoy such a luxury.

When my 15 minutes were up I got back on my feet, swung the pack onto my back and prepared myself for the last leg of Stage 1. The marking tape headed straight back into the jungle and just a few metres into it there was a hammock hanging between two trees that must have been for the checkpoint volunteers to relax in during their shift.

RACE DAY – STAGE 1

Lying on the ground next to it was one of the competitors, which surprised me because he hadn't passed through the checkpoint during the 15 minutes I had been resting there. That meant he must have been there longer than that. I asked him how he was doing and he said that soon after he had continued on from the checkpoint, he got very faint and started vomiting so he returned to the rest area to try and recover before continuing. He knew as well as I did that they were the classic signs of heat stress and I could tell from his body language that he was feeling pretty defeated. Although he was a fit and experienced ultra-endurance runner, he was from the UK so he wasn't used to running in such hot and humid conditions. He was in a safe place to be recovering though, so I wished him luck and continued on into the jungle.

The last section between checkpoint 4 and the finish line was the longest of Stage 1 and it included nearly 7km of more unforgiving climbs and descents before finally coming out onto the jungle road that passed through the village of Takuara, one of only three indigenous communities in the Flona. Local children greeted me as I emerged from the jungle track out onto the village road and their enthusiasm lifted my spirits as I high-fived them. While passing the few hundred metres through their village I was surprised to see a somewhat crude, but nonetheless functional, football field. There was no doubt that all Brazilians took their football very seriously, even in the remotest parts of the country!

After a grueling race time of 7 hours and 23 minutes I finally crossed the finish line for Stage 1, located in the village of Pini. The medics were set up under a sheltered area next to the village football field (it seems every village has one) and I parked myself on the grass next to it because I didn't want to have to walk another step more for now. I took my shoes, socks and long sleeved top off to help cool down before surrendering to the flat patch of grass beneath me.

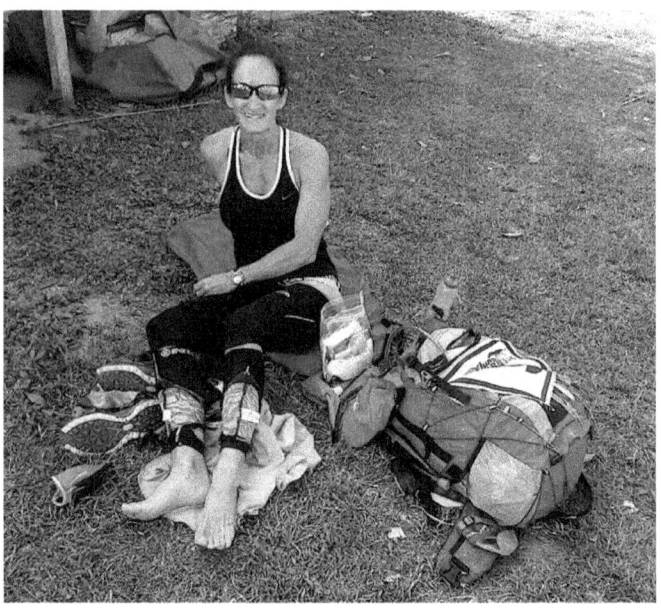

It was such a relief to lie down on my back, stretch my limbs out and feel the breeze on my skin. The muscles in my legs, back and neck were aching in quiet protest at what I had subjected them to and it was hard to focus on anything else. I wanted to mingle with the crowd and savor the glorious moment of completing Stage 1 but I just had to make do with observing the crowd from my supine position on the ground.

RACE DAY – STAGE 1

I was pleased to see that my feet were in good condition when I took my shoes and socks off, with no signs of blisters or damaged toenails. I had an enviable record of never having either had a blister or lost a toenail throughout the 4 years I had been running marathons, so was hoping to uphold the record through the Jungle Marathon. By all reports from previous year's events though, this record was going to be very difficult to maintain.

I continued with the my medical self-evaluation and determined that my stomach and head weren't showing any signs of heat stress, so I was feeling quietly confident that I would continue to cope with the climate challenges as I had hoped I would. I also had no cuts, insect bites or sunburn thanks to the protection my clothes gave me, so I was very pleased with my choice of race clothes and was happy to continue the event in the same manner.

My only problems were the muscle aches, which were causing me great discomfort but weren't life threatening or physically debilitating. The only solution was to try and decrease the weight in my backpack so it wasn't such a burden and while I thought I had only packed the bare essentials, I knew I had to be even more ruthless and remove all the dead weight I could find.

While still sitting on the ground, I grabbed my pack, up-ended it on the ground so everything was in front of me, and then commenced culling the what-I-thought-were-essential items from the absolute essentials.

I started with my food because I knew I would never eat more than a few spoonfuls of each packet given my absolute dislike of them. The casserole-type meals were not going to make the grade and only the macaroni cheese meals appealed. I emptied the contents of all the macaroni cheese sachets into a plastic bag so I could eliminate the weight and bulk of the thick foil pouches however, I kept one of them to use as a bowl to rehydrate and eat the food from.

Next to be culled were all the snacks I had packed which comprised mostly dried fruit products or sugary sweets. The super sweet taste of things like sultanas was too much for me, as were muesli bars and protein bars. While the extremely high sugar contents of these foods are a good energy source, they were just too sweet to be palatable. My stomach was craving food but only salty snacks, so my most treasured essentials were some small snack-sized packs of crisps. I only wished I had more of these instead of all the horrendous (taste-wise and cost wise!) dehydrated meals I had brought with me.

Once the food was sorted it was time to eliminate any non-essential clothing. As I was happy with the clothes I wore for the first day I decided to dump the spare set of race clothes and the spare camp clothes – one pair of knickers and a baggy T-shirt were going to have to get me through the evenings. The bikini and thongs (flip flops) stayed. The hat I could do without, as for the camera and my iPhone, which I had brought along as a spare camera. I had already streamlined all the mandatory medical and survival supplies before the start of the race so I couldn't afford to strip anything further from those. Unfortunately the bulkiest items were my hammock and rain sheet but there was nothing I could do about them as they had to stay.

After everything had been sorted into piles on the

RACE DAY – STAGE 1

ground I packed all the "keeper" items back into my pack. All the non-essential items were put into a spare dry sack and I gave those to Shirley, the race director, to store for me on the boat for the remainder of the race. Although I could now fit everything into my pack without having to hang things from the outside, it was still a tight squeeze to get the zip closed and the weight still felt like a heavy burden. It probably still weighed 10-12kg but it was the best I could do, so I would just have to live with it.

Unfortunately my work for the day wasn't done as I had to walk down to the camp site next to the river, which was about 200m away from where I was sitting, and hang my hammock up so I had a place to sleep. I didn't want to leave this task for too long because I didn't want to be doing it in the dark or have trouble finding spare trees to hang it from. Despite taking over 7 hours and 23 minutes to complete the 23km stage, there were still about 10 more people who were yet to complete the stage and I wanted to get my hammock hung before additional competition began vying for spots as well.

At the entrance to the camping area there were some local ladies at a makeshift drinks station who were handing out cups of cold fresh fruit juice made from Cupuacu, which is a tropical rainforest tree related to cacao. The juice is made from the white pulp of the fruit and it tastes like a combination of banana and pear. There was only enough for one cupful each and it's fresh taste left me longing for more.

I walked down to the campsite and found a spot to hang my hammock next to my Antarctic Marathon friends.

The camp was roughly segregated into Portuguese-speaking and English-speaking sections, although the entire area was so compact that no one was really very far from anyone else.

The river at this campsite was not very inviting but a quick dip in the murky water was desperately needed to wash away the day's accumulation of sweat, swamp and jungle muck. Although my race clothes desperately needed a dunk in the river as well, they were now dry on my body. Trying to get wet layers of tight lycra off is not an easy task at the best of times and, as it was unlikely they would have dried overnight, trying to pull on wet, clammy lycra the next morning would have been even harder. I decided washing could wait till the morning when the start of Stage 2 required us to swim across the river, and my panicky thrashing of arms and legs was sure to provide enough agitation to give them a good rinse.

After securing my hammock, I stripped off the layers of lycra, hung them along the hammock ties, put my bikini on and started walking bare-footed down the sandy riverbank towards the water. I hadn't gone very far before I felt the nipping of ants on my feet and I looked down to see the ground alive with them. I dashed back to my gear, slipped my shoes back on and headed back down again.

I left my shoes by the edge of the water and walked into the river just deep enough to be able to submerge my whole body in the hope that I would feel better for doing so. After what I had been through in Stage 1, this murky river water was a welcome relief and even the threat of piranhas couldn't deter me from enjoying the buoyant effects the water was having on my weary body. There was a young Brazilian guy already down there doing the same thing. Although we spoke different languages we managed to communicate, via exaggerated facial expressions, a mutual appreciation for the therapeutic effect the water was having on our bodies.

As good as the water felt, it was hard to ignore the slimy mud under my feet. There was no nice white sand at this campsite, just rotting vegetation and silty sludge lining the shallow waters along the river's edge. The support crew's riverboat was moored alongside where I was bathing, with the wooden gangplank stretching from the deck down to the water's edge.

The race director and her team of Brazilian helpers slept on this boat and, together with everyone's spare luggage, it carried all the drinking and cooking water to each campsite. It was off limits to the race competitors and despite its old and crude bathroom and kitchen facilities, it was luxurious compared to what we had in the camps.

This would be the fourth night of sleeping in my hammock and I was hoping my exhausted state would help me fall into a deeper and longer sleep than what I'd been able to achieve over the previous 3 nights. The amount of sand was building up in the bottom of my hammock but I was starting to get used to ignoring it when I first lay down, despite it getting trapped between my sweaty skin and the nylon fabric that wrapped around me. It felt like I was trapped inside a moth's cocoon all night however, instead of emerging as a beautifully transformed creature in the morning, I only flopped out as a smellier, more disheveled version of the person I had been the night before.

Upon returning to the campsite, the American husband

and wife team were setting up their hammocks next to mine. The husband was the man I had seen at checkpoint 3 with the red face, so I was glad to see they had both made it to the end of Stage 1. They explained how they had met up with the Welsh guy, Lee, who I had passed while he was recovering from heat stress near checkpoint 4 and, despite his extended rest, he was once again struggling to stay on his feet. It was clear when they found him that he would not have been able to support both his body weight and the weight of his backpack.

They convinced him to drop his pack to give him a better chance of being able to walk with them to the finish line where he could get medical aid. The support crew "sweepers" would be able to collect his bag off the track when they came through at the end of the day, as they would do at the end of each day throughout the race, to make sure no one was left stranded on the track.

When the three of them made it to the finish line Lee presented to the medic station with serious heat stress and his condition quickly deteriorated. The doctors immediately administered intravenous fluids to him as he contorted in pain on the ground, with his whole body appearing to cramp up. In true reality TV style, the film crew captured every agonizing moment of Lee's medical intervention. I have no doubt the scene will be prime trailer footage for their documentary when it eventually goes to air.

This would mark the end to Lee's 7-day endurance attempt but he aimed to rest up for the next couple of days and hope that he would be recovered and acclimatized enough to compete in the Stage 4 stand-alone 42km marathon distance event.

RACE DAY – STAGE 1

Yoshi, the Japanese competitor, crossed the finish line in a race time of 8 hours 34 minutes – still dressed in his cow suit! I couldn't believe he had done the entire stage in the heavy suit, through stream and swamp crossings and up and down the grueling climbs and descents. This guy was a machine. He should have melted inside all that suffocating furry material. He had apparently also recently completed the Marathon des Sables in the same suit. Although this was an extraordinary feat, the 7-day ultra marathon through the Sahara Desert doesn't expose competitors to the extreme humidity or terrain that the Jungle Marathon does, so everyone was quietly expecting the Amazon conditions to take their toll on him. He was to prove us all wrong – on day one at least.

Despite the communication barrier, Yoshi made friends with the local children while passing through their village when he stopped and pulled a bottle of bubble-making liquid out of his cow suit and proceeded to blow bubbles at the excited kids. Despite being physically and mentally exhausted, he still made time to show his appreciation to the local village people who cheered us on as we shuffled past their primitive homes. He may not have been the fittest person in the Jungle Marathon but he clearly had a heart bigger than everyone else combined. A photo snapped by the race photographer as he reached the finish line of Stage 1 shows him flanked by a large crowd of excited children who accompanied him along the last stretch of road into the village. He may not have been the first person to cross the finish line that day but he was definitely the winner in the eyes of these children.

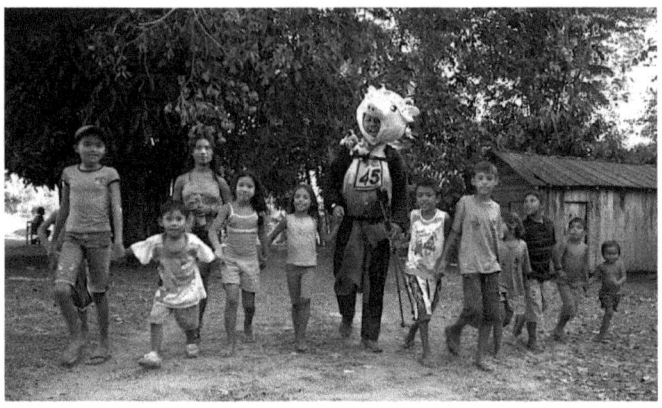

The first person to cross the finish line for Stage 1 was Austrian competitor Bernard, who completed it in an incredible race time of 2 hours 51 minutes. I've got no idea how it was humanly possible to complete that course in such a time. It's truly amazing what the human body is capable of when well trained. Trail running requires, and further develops, a fitness base like no other sport, with the leg strength and cardiovascular fitness of these elite athletes being a testament to that. With most of my running being done on city roads or treadmills, I knew the extreme terrain and climate of the Amazon Jungle would push my body to its limits and day one had just lived up to my expectations.

The final competitor to complete Stage 1, with a race time of 9 hours 24 minutes, got to the camp just as the last glimpses of daylight disappeared. With everyone present and accounted for it was time for an assembly to discuss what lay ahead of us on Stage 2 of the Jungle Marathon.

Although the distance we would have to cover was to be

slightly longer than today's stage, the terrain would fortunately be much less extreme. The day would start off with a swim of approximately 150m across the river before traversing 24km of flat or undulating tracks through the jungle and then finish with a few kilometres along the sandy road leading into the village of Tauri.

To hear that there would be none of the steep climbs that we had to endure for Stage 1 was music to my ears. I had no idea how my body would be feeling after a night sleeping. I was concerned that the punishment I had put it through today could produce an unprecedented bout of delayed onset muscle soreness in spiteful revenge. All I knew was that I wanted to maximize the amount of time I could lie in my hammock with the weight off my legs and back. This would give my metabolism the best possible chance of restoring vital glycogen supplies to my muscles and eliminating the lactate by-product of todays grueling workout.

After forcing myself to eat a small amount of reconstituted macaroni cheese I retired to my hammock and hoped that the aching pain in my back wouldn't stop me from getting to sleep. I fully expected to only get intermittent sleep but I was happy to settle for that, knowing that I would still clock up at least 8 hours of restorative time off my feet.

Stage 1 Race Summary

254km – Male

Bernard Plessberger (Austria) was the first to cross the finish line in an impressive time of just 2:51:18, with Brazilian Marcelo Sinoca not far behind him, in a time of 3:06:38. Third was Hirofumi Ono (Japan) in a time of 3:15:22.

Yoshi (The Cow) Yokoyama (Japan) was the last of the 254km male competitors to finish in a time of 8:34:02 but considering he was wearing a big thick cow suit for the entire race he put in an incredible performance.

A total of three runners in this category suffered considerably in the hot and humid conditions and were unable to attempt Stage 2 or 3 due to heat stress, but they hoped to recover fully to be able to complete the 42km marathon distance of Stage 4.

Of the original 37 starters in the male category there would be 34 continuing on to Stage 2.

254km – Female

Jacqueline Terto (Brazil) was the first women to cross the finish line in a time of 4:52:39. Jacqui is a past champion of the Jungle Marathon, having won the 254km event twice before and the 127km event once. She had given herself a good starting lead in this years event and would definitely have a great chance of winning the race.

The second female over the line was Marie Ann Danet (France) also in a remarkable time of 5:18:29. My finishing time of 7:23:07 made me the third 254km female competitor over the line although the 6 females from the

127km event all finished ahead of me.

Kim Frankish (UK) was the next of the 254km women to finish in a time of 8:31:30. Kim had previously completed the famed Marathon des Sables, a multi-stage ultra-endurance race through the Sahara Desert, so she knew what she had to do to survive the grueling distances of the Jungle Marathon.

Sandy Simons was originally a competitor in the 254km event but her husband, Fred, was struggling to survive the hot and humid conditions and was forced to pull out of Stage 2 and 3 so she also decided not to continue.

Jacquie Palmer (USA) was the last of the women to finish Stage 1 in a time of 9:24:02. Jacquie was returning as a competitor this year after attending the 2012 Jungle Marathon as a volunteer. Her determination was to be tested to its limits as she continued through the next 5 stages of the race. The later the competitors get back to the camp each night, the less sleep and recovery time they have before the start of the next stage, so sleep deprivation starts to play a big role as the stages get longer in distance.

127km – Male

Out of the 10 competitors for the 4-stage event the first to finish Stage 1 was Lucas Antonio Marques (Brazil) in a time of 3:32:28. Second across the line was Themos Sgouras (Greece) in a time of 4:20:21 and following in third place was Caio Tarantino (Brazil) in 4:57:20. The remaining seven runners were spread out in the field, with the last crossing the finish line in 8:07:46.

127km – Women

Of the six women competing in this category the first over the line was Andreia Henssler (Brazil) in a time of 4:22:02, closely followed by Stefanie Bacon (UK) in 4:32:29. Andreia and Stefanie were the first women to cross the finish line out of both the 254km and 127km events in the very tough first stage.

Carol Barcello, the journalist from TV Globo, also put in a strong performance with a finishing time of 5:49:51 - even with the handicaps of stopping to help an injured runner and signing autographs!

Fourth over the line was Anna Chernova (Russia) who also lost some time throughout the stage when helping the injured runner. Her time of 6:01:11 was nearly half an hour ahead of Danielle Whitney, an American who now resides in the UK, and Karen Curtis, an Australian ex-pat who now resides in the USA, who crossed the finish line together.

Chapter 6

RACE DAY – STAGE 2

Pini to Tauri – Approximately 24km

Stage 2 Brief

Start (Pini) to Checkpoint 1: 6.60km
Checkpoint 1 to Checkpoint 2: 6.14km
Checkpoint 2 to Checkpoint 3: 5.14km
Checkpoint 3 to Finish (Tauri): 6.10km

There will be a compulsory 15 minute break at each checkpoint

---

Awakening to the pre-dawn cockal-doodle-doo'ing of the village roosters was now a part of everyone's morning routine. Every village in the Amazon Jungle seemed to have an ample supply of roosters and dogs. I could only guess that the reason they kept the starving, mangy dogs around their homes was to warn of possible threats, although most of them seemed so weak and docile that I doubt they would have been capable of even raising a bark.

Once I was conscious enough to remember where I was and what I had been through the day before, I started moving my limbs to test for any possible damage before attempting to stand on my feet. Initial responses were encouraging and I was quietly confident there was no damage that would prevent me from continuing with Stage 2. I scrambled out of my hammock and shuffled quietly around the other hammocks to go to the "bathroom" before preparing some food for breakfast. It was then time to change into the cold, damp and smelly race clothes that had been airing out overnight but had not dried in the humid jungle air. They only felt disgusting for a few minutes while they warmed up to my body temperature, by which time my nose had become accustomed to the smell as well.

Although I didn't know it at the time, there were three competitors who would be unable to continue due to the heat stress they had suffered the previous day. Along with Lee from Wales, there was also an Argentinian runner, Rene, who failed to finish Stage 1. Although the American, Fred, had completed the stage he had a restless night with bouts of vomiting and was too weak to be able to start Stage 2. All three would rest for the next two days and compete in the 42km marathon stage on day 4.

During the race briefing the night before we had been told that after the initial river crossing we would not have any further water encounters on day 2. We were advised that if we wanted to keep our feet dry for as long as possible then it would be wise to carry our shoes and socks in our dry sack while crossing the river and put them back on afterwards.

Running with wet feet greatly increases the chances of getting blisters so you really want to avoid it if possible. I slid my backpack, shoes and socks into the large waterproof dry sack and folded the top over a few times

RACE DAY – STAGE 2

before snapping the buckle shut. The trapped air inside the sack provided the added value of buoyancy, enabling the bundle to act as a flotation device and assisting me while paddling across the river.

The only problem with having my shoes in the sack was that while we were waiting on the riverbank for the race to begin my feet were at the mercy of the ants. I shifted my weight from one foot to the other like I was doing some crazy Amazon riverbank dance, hoping that there wasn't a bullet ant amongst them.

It was easy to pick the serious, experienced ultra marathon runners from the novice, fun-run competitors like myself, because they all kept their backpack on their back and their shoes and socks on their feet. Every minute counted with these competitors and they weren't going to be slowed down by having to muck around with their gear every time they crossed a bit of water.

I weighed up the pros and cons and have to admit I was worried about whether I could swim 150m across a deep river with a heavy backpack on my back. I was relieved to see that the majority of the competitors had stuffed their pack into a dry sack and were lining up on the riverbank in bare feet like me. Given my total lack of experience at this type of event, I was relying on my observations of everyone else to act as my guide.

To say I was getting anxious about having to swim across the river would be an understatement. Wallowing in the shallow waters edge was one thing. Swimming out into the middle of a river that was most likely infested with piranhas and countless other creatures, was a whole different story.

I tried to calm my nerves by reassuring myself that I would have plenty of people ahead of me thrashing their arms and legs about, which would hopefully warn the aquatic life of impending danger and scare them into fleeing the scene. Apparently race support crew members had spotted dozens of caiman in the river just next to the start line late in the evening while the runners were sleeping, but thankfully I didn't know this at the time. I'm sure the race director did her best to keep this bit of information quiet so we wouldn't be even more freaked out than we already were.

As the countdown to the start drew closer one of the medics swam out into the middle of the river, staying close to the rope that had been stretched from one side of the river to the other. There were known non-swimmers amongst the competitors and the rope would act as a safeguard for those who weren't confident of their ability to swim across the river.

As the vulnerable lone female medic swam closer to the middle of the river through murky water I was feeling nervous just watching. I felt like I was watching a scene from a pop culture thriller movie and at any moment she would be violently yanked under the water, her arms flailing above her head in desperation as she took her last breath of air before disappearing into the depths of the deadly river. I wondered if she had drawn the short straw when deciding who would act as the sacrificial lamb and be the first to test the waters, or if she willingly volunteered. I was so glad it wasn't me!

Two Brazilian bombeiros joined the medic in the water as the drone camera whizzed overhead in preparation to record footage of the flurry of arms and legs that would soon be disturbing the tranquil dawn sunrise over the river. With the support crew in place, it was time to start Stage 2. Shirley began counting down from 10 to 1 in Portuguese as everyone made their way to the edge of the water.

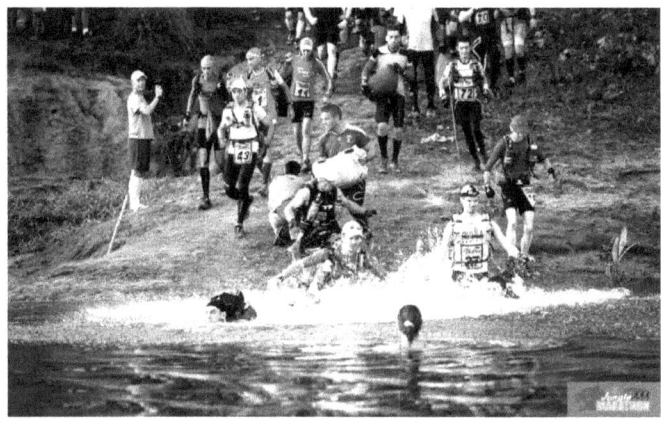

The ensuing excitement and yahooing all but smothered my dread of the thought of running into the water fully clothed and to my surprise, once my body was fully submerged up to my neck, it actually felt quite pleasant. I had subconsciously braced to be hit by cold water but the water temperature was virtually the same as the air temperature, which enabled a shock-free transition from the riverbank into the river.

As I quickly adjusted and relaxed into the swim, I decided not to try and use the rope because it had become submerged as dozens of hands grabbed hold of it and used it to pull themselves along. My dry sack was very buoyant and made me feel quite safe so I just held it out in front of me and kicked my legs until I got close to the riverbank on the other side.

The embankment was quite muddy so I grabbed hold of the rope, used it to help pull myself out of the water and then quickly moved out of the way as soon as I got my footing so I didn't hold up anybody emerging behind me. The elite competitors took off out of the water and up the riverbank without missing a beat, whereas everyone else spread out and unpacked their gear from their dry sack and put their shoes and socks on before following the race marker tape into the dense jungle beyond the river.

The non-swimmers stayed at the back of the pack so the race support crew could help them if they needed it. Vicky, the race medic stationed in the middle of the river, saw one of the female competitors go under the water so she raced towards her and brought her back up to the surface. Unfortunately the panic-stricken lady then pushed Vicki under the water which left both of them in need of rescuing. The bombeiro saw what was happening, quickly raced over and helped the competitor over to the other side of the river.

A system was then worked out to help the non-swimmers, with Vicky towing them to half way and then the bombeiro taking them the rest of the way. They worked in relay until they got everyone across. Fortunately Yoshi, who was also a non-swimmer, didn't wear his cow suit for the crossing and wisely chose to put it on only once he was clear of the water.

Once my shoes and socks were back on my feet, I rolled up the dry sack and stuffed it into one of the outside

RACE DAY – STAGE 2

pockets on my backpack. It felt nice to have dry socks on my feet and I was feeling pretty good as I jogged away from the riverbank and into the jungle.

The feeling of contentment was to be very short-lived though as I had only travelled a few hundred metres before being faced with a shallow stream. I stopped dead in disbelief and thought "You've got to be kidding me!" and contemplated my next move. The choices were to waste more time taking my shoes and socks off or just run through it and accept that my feet would be wet for the whole stage.

I couldn't be bothered undressing again so after a few seconds of deliberation I ploughed through the shallow water and continued on my way. Stewing over the fact that we had been told there would be no more water after the river crossing wasn't going to help me so I laughed it off and made a mental note not to believe everything Shirley tells us in the briefings!

The 6.6km to checkpoint 1 was mainly along flat jungle tracks, which was a welcomed relief after the previous days tortuous hills. Although the ground was flat, there were plenty of tripping obstacles to watch out for in addition to keeping an eye on the route marker tape. We had been reminded of the dangers of knife-sharp plants in this area and also an abundance of snakes, so it was important to stay vigilant and pay close attention to where you placed your feet and hands.

Although I had no serious muscle soreness from the previous day my legs felt quite heavy and my upper back ached under the weight of my backpack, so I alternated jogging and walking to try and keep moving as quickly as I could. I was surprised to catch up to the two Norwegians Berndt and Petter and we continued on to the checkpoint together. They had a cameraman travelling with them who was documenting their race so I dropped behind the two runners as they ran on ahead so I didn't spoil the shot of them giving their cameraman a victorious wave as they ran into the checkpoint.

Like the first day, we were required to wait a compulsory 15 minutes at checkpoints today, but I desperately longed for a break so I didn't need a race rule to convince me of resting. I took my pack off and lay down flat on my back for several minutes.

I knew that any amount of time wasn't going to be long enough to make me feel good while I had the pack to carry, so I figured I just had to get back up and keep moving towards the finish line as quickly as I could. After topping up my water supplies, I signaled to the medics that I was good to go and they ticked my name off their list as I continued on my way.

The Norwegians left the checkpoint a few minutes ahead of me so I was on my own again as I followed the marker tape off the dirt road and back into the jungle. Checkpoint 2 was approximately 6km away and I was hoping it would all be on relatively flat ground. My mind was still haunted by the hill climbs and descents of the day before and I was in no hurry to go through that pain again, although I knew I would have to eventually.

The jungle was very peaceful and the assortment of birdcalls was keeping me entertained, especially the one that sounded like a wolf whistle. Every time I heard it I would smile at the thought of beautiful jungle birds sitting on branches and whistling at the women as they ran past – just like construction workers do when you're running through city streets!

I was mostly walking now as the running took too much of a toll on my aching back and legs. I forced myself into a steady cadence as I tried to cover the distance as quickly as I could. It was impossible keeping my mind off my aching body, but without the company of others to distract me I found it hard to remain focused on anything else.

This changed though when I felt an unexpected very sharp sting on my leg and realized that something had bitten me through my tights. I instinctively slapped the spot with my hand before even looking to see what was causing the pain. Just as I did I felt more bites on both my legs and I frantically started slapping my thighs with both my hands however, as I did I noticed the offending insects were biting my hands as well! I realized that I must have been next to a nest of wasps so I sprinted off down the track, slapping my legs as I ran in an effort to stop the attack. It seemed that every time I got a bite on one of my legs and slapped at the offending wasp, I would then receive a bite on my hand from the same wasp in retaliation. The attack continued for several seconds as I sprinted down the track, frantically slapping at my arms and legs like a crazy women until the biting finally stopped. The adrenalin jolt to my body in response to the attack was immense and I marveled later about the human body's incredible "flight or fight response" – one moment I was struggling to find the energy to put one foot in front of the other and the next I was sprinting through the jungle at a speed I never knew I was capable of!

Once the biting stopped and the threat had passed, I stopped to catch my breath and assess the damage. I had several bites on my legs and several on the palms of my hands and they all stung like hell. The pain was intense and I had no idea how long it would continue for. I was hoping it wouldn't be as long or as bad as what Shirley had to endure with the bullet ant bite. Fortunately, within a few minutes the intensity of the pain started to decrease and I continued walking. The pain died off after another 10 minutes and I breathed a sigh of relief once I was confident there were no lasting effect from the stings. I certainly hoped there would be no other surprise attacks like that waiting for me further down the track but I knew there was a good chance it could happen again at any time. Now I had to watch out for trips, snakes, marker tape...*and wasps!*

As I made my way along the jungle track I alternated my attention between watching my feet for tripping hazards and snakes and watching the trees for pieces of marker tape to make sure I didn't wander off the race route. The undergrowth here wasn't as dense as what it had been on the Stage 1 route, so rather than having one well defined track there was more of an anastomosing network of possible tracks heading in the same direction. I guessed that either the local people or wild animals had formed the roughly defined paths while doing whatever it is they do out here.

Sometimes the marker tape wasn't always visible and I'd just keep walking hoping to pick it up again. I thought I was still heading in the right direction until I suddenly got a feeling of déjà vu when some of the trees started to look familiar. There were occasional fallen trees to step over and it was one of these that sparked a subconscious alarm bell in my mind. I had an uneasy feeling about the path I was taking, but then I saw another piece of marker tape so guessed it was all in my imagination.

As I continued on past another few pieces of marker tape I still couldn't quell the weird feeling that something wasn't quite right however, I brushed it off and reasoned that if I was passing pieces of tape then I must be on the right track. That lasted until I came face-to-face with the group of Americans approaching from the opposite direction! In that instant I finally figured out what my subconscious mind had been trying to tell me – I had somehow been turned around 180 degrees and was now heading back the way I had come from!

Arrgghh! More wasted time and energy that I couldn't afford to lose. I had no idea how I managed to do it but after getting over the frustration I was grateful that at least my wrong turn didn't leave me lost in the jungle. I guessed I must have only been backtracking for a few minutes and reckoned I hadn't really lost too much time.

Now that I had some company I felt a lot safer and I figured that with five sets of eyes watching out for marker tape I had a better chance of not straying off the track again. Danielle, Jason and Karen were the Americans I had met while competing in the Antarctic Ice Marathon nearly a year before and the 4th person was Danielle's partner Ed, who was from the UK where Danielle now lives. The five of us pushed on through the jungle until we finally reached checkpoint 2.

Just as we walked into the rest area and had our names recorded by the medics, we all noticed the French competitor, Marie, walking towards us from the opposite side of the checkpoint. I was wondering why she was approaching from the other direction and the medics were also looking bewildered until Marie asked them if this was checkpoint 3. As soon as the words came out of her mouth her face mirrored the dawning horror of what the medics were about to tell her: "This is checkpoint 2 and you left here about an hour ago!"

She had done exactly the same thing I had done only she wasn't lucky enough to run into people coming the other way, so had no idea she was heading back in the wrong direction. She was mentally and physically shattered. She looked like she was going to collapse from shock and I felt devastated for her, thinking that if it had happened to me I don't know if I would have had the strength to continue. As well as being physically exhausted she looked to be suffering from heat stress and knew she couldn't immediately continue on. When the Americans and I left the checkpoint, Marie was still there and she would end up spending another few hours resting before continuing on to complete the stage, nearly three hours after we had crossed the finish line.

The last two sections between checkpoints 2, 3 and the finish line covered over 11km of jungle tracks and dirt roads leading into the village of Tauri. I kept pace with the group of four friends and was grateful for their company, feeling the safety that being in a group provided. My hopeless sense of direction had already failed me twice in as many days and I didn't want to risk putting it to the test again by being in the jungle alone.

RACE DAY – STAGE 2

I crossed the finish line for Stage 2 in a time of 5 hours 44 minutes. The 24km trekked felt very much longer and I couldn't help but compare the time it normally takes me to run a road half marathon of 21.1km, about 1 hour 50 minutes. The extra burden of a heavy backpack, combined with the extreme terrain and often soft ground, meant it was impossible to make time estimates before each stage of the race. All I could hope for was to get to each campsite before sunset because there was no way I wanted to be stuck out in the jungle after dark.

Although my legs, back and neck ached immensely, I was feeling better than I did when I finished Stage 1 the day before, so I went straight to the campsite and found some trees to hang my hammock from. The sky had by then become very dark and it looked like a tropical storm was about to provide a break from the usual afternoon heat and humidity. I raced to get my hammock and rain sheet hung up so I could store my gear under the cover they would provide. I had only just completed the task when the heavens opened up and delivered a 30-minute deluge that had everyone racing for the cover of the two concrete shelter areas in the village we were staying at.

The rain cooled me down but the accompanying wind made me feel very cold. The rain dropped the air temperature considerably and my exhausted body was having trouble coping. I cowered in one of the sheltered areas trying to stay out of the wind but the structure didn't have fully enclosed walls so the wind and rain were able to penetrate part of the way inside. I started to get concerned that the showers might continue into the night and I'd have to go to bed wet but fortunately this wasn't to happen. The deluge soaked the ground beneath our hammocks but the sandy soil prevented the area from turning into a muddy quagmire, for which I was extremely grateful.

The village of Tauri was similar to the one we had stayed in the night before. The primitive huts and concrete sheltered common areas were nestled between the dirt access road and the banks of the Tapajos River. This camping area had a few more facilities though, with two "toilets" that looked to be permanent structures situated to the right of the track leading into the area where our hammocks were hanging. These toilets were still just holes in the ground that you had to squat over, but at least they had four walls around them and lockable doors!

The bigger of the two cement sheltered areas was set up as the medic's station and the other was used as a makeshift kitchen. I was ecstatic to see a variety of local dishes laid out on a big table with paper plates next to them but was soon to discover that the food was only for the people who were planning to do just the Stage 4 one day marathon. The ultra marathon competitors were still only allowed to eat whatever food they had in their backpacks. Oh how cruel! We did however, get treated to a cup of freshly made cupuaca juice again that the local village people had prepared. Although it tasted a bit strange at first, I devoured the cupful in seconds as my body craved the luxury of a drink that was more than just water or electrolytes.

The river was about 50m away from the medic's hut and looked very similar to where we had camped the previous night. The banks were littered with leaves and stones which provided cover for the multitude of insects and reptiles that call the jungle floor their home. The ants continued to pose a threat to unsuspecting bare feet so I kept my shoes on while exploring the riverbank. I was still trying to thaw out following my wind-chilled soaking so thought I'd pass on a recovery swim in the river, fearing that when I got out of the water I'd have trouble warming up again.

I returned to my hammock to change from my running clothes into my camp T-shirt and knickers, both of which were getting very smelly now. I could have washed them but they would not have been able to dry during the day while I was running and I wanted to keep them dry at all costs. Smelly clothes are bearable for sleeping in – wet ones are not! Fortunately everyone had the same problem so I think our noses were desensitized to the point that our brains just ignored it.

While I was changing out of my wet clothes I heard someone yelling out from the direction of the medic's hut and curious people started to head towards the area to see what the commotion was about. It turned out that after two days of running through the jungle the Greek competitor, Themos, had presented to the medics with 5 big blisters on his feet. Much to his horror the doctors treated them with dreaded "Hot Shots", a common procedure the U.S. military use to treat blisters.

The hot shot is performed by first draining the fluid from the blister and then injecting the same amount of compound tincture of benzoin (Friar's Balsam). This helps seal the space created by the blister, serves as a local antiseptic, and prevents further abrasion or loss of skin.

They became known as a "hot shot" amongst military personnel due to the extreme burning sensation that is experienced for several moments after the tincture is applied.

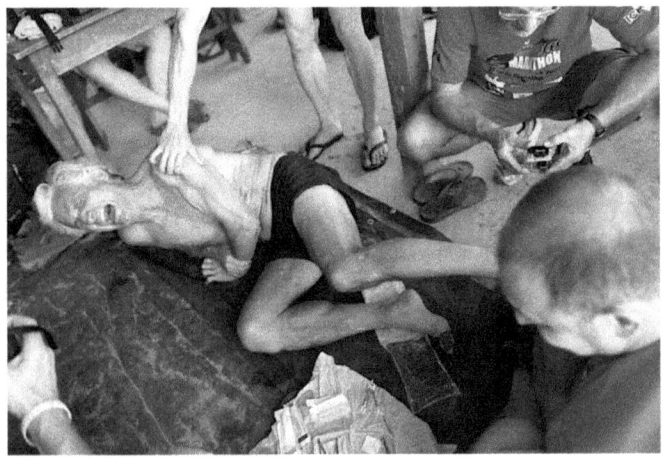

Themos' agonizing screams were testament to the amount of pain these injections cause and he soon had a large audience of village people, competitors, volunteers and cameramen watching and filming his ordeal. I'm sure his screams would have been music to the film crew's ears as they captured the gritty reality of life as a Jungle Marathoner. I'm pretty sure no-one else volunteered for a hot shot after that day!

Nearly three hours after I had finished Stage 2 the Japanese competitor, Yoshi, crossed the finish line. He arrived in the camp without his cow suit, wearing just a T-shirt and underwear and sporting a long, deep graze up the left side of his thigh.

RACE DAY – STAGE 2

Carol, the journalist from TV Globo, helped him offload his backpack while people fussed around him, trying to get him to go to the medics to look at his wound. He appeared to be quite dazed and the communication barrier didn't help matters as people tried to figure out what had happened to him. Considering Stage 2 was quite tame in regards to terrain compared to the previous day, it was hard to imagine how he had ended up in the state he was in. The effects on his body must have been more serious than just the visible grazes on his leg, as he would not compete in the following 3 stages of the competition. Yoshi, it seems, was yet another victim of the debilitating jungle heat and humidity.

Once I had changed into my dry T-shirt, I took advantage of the complimentary massage offered by one of the two Brazilian women who were in the camps each day to attend to the aching bodies of the competitors. Before the massage even began, I was already languishing in the joy of being able to lie down on a firm, flat bed for the first time in five days and wished I could have stayed there all night. The massage only added to the delight of the experience, although the fine grit on my skin that was massaged through with the oil felt a bit unpleasant at first however, I soon accepted it for the unique jungle massage experience that it was.

Everyone had completed Stage 2 and was in the camp relaxing by late afternoon, so Shirley called an assembly to brief us on the events of the day and then outline what to expect the following day during Stage 3.

One of the highlights of the evening briefing sessions

was when Shirley handed out any email messages that competitors received via the Jungle Marathon website in the previous 24 hours. Friends and family were able to keep in touch by sending messages, which the race organizers printed out each day and gave to the runners.

An interesting email came through for the person who was wearing race number 48 from the person who had worn this number in the previous years race. His message was to wish him luck and that if he survived Stage 3 then he would be home and hosed. Upon hearing this I began to feel anxious about what the next day held in store for us and wondered if I could survive it. Our bodies were already worn down, both physically and mentally, from the two days of racing we had already completed but the distance to be covered for Stage 3 was a grueling 14km further than what we had covered in either Stage 1 or 2.

Stage 3 would start again with a river crossing and then take us deep into the jungle. Steep climbs and descents would again test us. The route would also be passing through the areas of jungle that had the highest jaguar populations, so we were warned to be vigilant. The stage would finish at a deep jungle campsite around which armed guards were to be patrolling at night to keep the jaguars away. I was willing to bet that by the end of the Stage 3, I would be praying for a jaguar to put me out of my misery!

With the briefing completed, Shirley revealed that there was still plenty of the cupuaca juice left over. She organized for it to be brought out to the table where I was sitting and I helped pour it into small plastic cups. It was like a feeding frenzy as people jostled to grab a cup of the nutritious juice. It was very warm by now and the taste wasn't anything special but that didn't stop the wonderful fresh food from being devoured. By that point, anything that wasn't rehydrated was truly a gift from the heavens and I knew my body desperately needed the calories and nutrition the juice provided.

My inability to palate the dehydrated meals was now becoming a major concern. As already described, the only variety of which I could force even a few spoonfuls down was the macaroni cheese. I was having this for breakfast and dinner but I could only stand a small amount before I would find myself gagging on it. I still had a few sweet snacks, like dried fruit, but I could only stomach a small amount of these as well. My most cherished food remained the small variety snack packs of salty crisps but unfortunately I only had enough for one small pack a day, so I had to ration them out.

The local village people mingled amongst the runners and the children took delight in the attention they received. The people here seemed to be a bit more westernized in their style of clothing. The young girls wore pretty dresses and had beautiful smiling faces that seemed to camouflage the reality of their primitive existence in the jungle. It was such a world away from the lives most of the competitors lead.

Experiencing these places first hand certainly makes you appreciate your comfortable life in the civilized world and not to take it for granted. In saying that it still doesn't make me want to pack a tent and go camping on the weekends. While experiences like this trip are educational, thought provoking and amazing, I would definitely be lying if I said it was enjoyable. Give me a hot shower and the fresh sheets of a hotel bed any day!

Despite the persistent muscle pain in my upper back and shoulders I was faring pretty well. I still had no signs of blisters or any damage to my feet and my long sleeved and legged clothing had done a great job of protecting my skin from rough plants and the weather. The heat and humidity had not had any serious effects on me, with no signs of heat stress or dehydration. I just had to hope that I could continue like this for another 5 days!

Stage 2 Race Summary

254km – Male

Bernard (Austria), was the first over the line again in a time of 2:33:36, with Marcelo (Brazil), very close behind him in 2:35:21. Sousa Fredlsen (Brazil) was third over the line in 2:54:18 just ahead of Hiro (Japan), who crossed the finish line in 2:57:02.

The remaining 254km male competitors were well spread out with the last, Yoshi the cow, taking 8:18:13 to finish the stage.

254km – Female

Brazilian Jacquie was considerably stronger than the rest of the field and crossed the finish line in an impressive time of 4:08:08. I was the next to cross in a time of 5:44:02. Marie lost a lot of time, energy and motivation after taking a wrong turn and ended up finishing the stage with Kim (UK) and Jacquie (US) in a time of 8:28:01.

RACE DAY – STAGE 2

127km – Male

Lucas Marques (Brazil) put in another winning performance to be first over the finish line in a time of 3:05:22, nearly an hour ahead of the second place getter Themos (Greece) who finished in 3:53:10. Caio (Brazil) only just made it across the line before Clayton Conservani, from TV Globo, who crossed in 4:05:38. The remaining 127km males followed with the last competitor finishing in a time of 6:53:47.

127km – Women

Andreia (Brazil) was again too strong for Stefanie Bacon and finished in 3:47:36 to Stephanie's 4:04:05. A very close third place, in a time of 4:05:35, was Carol Barcello who was able to put in a solid performance during this stage with no interruptions like in Stage 1. Anna Chernova was only a few minutes behind Carol in a time of 4:10:00 and Danielle Whitney and Karen Curtis triumphantly crossing the finish line in 5:43:48 and 5:43:58.

Of the 254km male competitors who ran Stage 2 only Yoshi from Japan, would be unable to tackle Stage 3 the next day. He would be the fourth to pull out since the start of the race. There was one male from the 127km runners who would not be able to continue any further stages.

All of the 254km and 127km women who completed Stage 2 would line up for the start of Stage 3 the next morning.

Chapter 7

RACE DAY – STAGE 3

Tauri to Deep Jungle Camp – 38km

Stage 3 Brief

Start (Tauri) to Checkpoint 1 (Nazare): 3.76km
Checkpoint 1 to Checkpoint 2: 6.70km
Checkpoint 2 to Checkpoint 3: 8,31km
Checkpoint 3 to Checkpoint 4 (Marituba): 11.95km
Checkpoint 4 to Finish (Piquiatuba): 7.15km

Stage 3 was to be a much longer distance than what we had covered in the previous two stages, so we needed to start before sunrise to make the most of the available daylight. The village roosters never failed to wake us up in plenty of time to get up and be ready for the start of the race each day. They had become our reliable jungle alarm clocks.

I lay in my hammock for a while after waking, taking stock of how my body was feeling and considering what lay ahead in today's stage. Unlike yesterday morning, I wasn't anxious about the river crossing we had to do at the start because I knew what to expect now. The river crossing start for Stage 2 proved to be less terrifying than expected and I held onto the thought of how nice and warm the water felt once I was swimming across. This morning's swim would be over 100m further than yesterday's but I felt confident of being able to swim the necessary 250m without too much of a problem.

The thought of swimming hundreds of metres across the murky brown waters of a caiman and piranha-infested Amazonian tributary is terrifying but doing anything in your life, especially for the first time, can be scary. It was comforting to finally have that experience under my belt. As an aside, I was later to find out that Joao, one of the competitors from Brazil, had brought his swimming goggles because he was curious to watch the aquatic life in that part of the Amazon and came face to face with the "mother of all piranhas." Ignorance is bliss I say!

After checking for ants, spiders and scorpions in my shoes and finding them free of any threat, I slipped my feet into them while sitting in my hammock. Most people were already up and about and refueling on their rehydrated breakfast meals.

I made a trip to the toilet first, which by now was getting very smelly. I alternated between holding my breath and breathing through my mouth in an attempt to avoid the overpowering stench of human faeces as I awkwardly squatted over the annoyingly small hole in the ground. Every time I was faced with executing this task it made me realize how mankind's natural development of being able to sit in a squat position has been compromised by the invention of the chair. An action that is perfectly normal and comfortable for a toddler or "uncivilized" indigenous person has now become an uncomfortable and strenuous position for a westernized adult. Yet another reason why I hate camping.

With the morning ablutions out of the way I prepared a small amount of macaroni cheese, along with some sweet dried fruit snacks, for breakfast. I filled my drink bladder and water bottle from the large bottles of supplied water and made my way back to my hammock to start packing up my gear.

The cold, damp and smelly race clothes had been hanging over my hammock ropes all night but were no drier now than when I took them off last night. The tropical air was too humid to draw any moisture out of my clothes so pulling the tight, wet lycra layers on was an uncomfortable process. Fortunately it only took a minute for the cold clothes to heat up to my body temperature and then they didn't feel too bad.

Although I planned to have my shoes and socks in my dry sack while I swam across the river, I put them on so I would have some protection from the ants while we were waiting for the race to start. My only luxury for the whole week was the clean pair of socks I would start each stage in. Even though they didn't stay dry for very long, I still cherished the moment the dry fabric would hug my feet each morning. Events like this certainly make you appreciate the little things in life.

Quite a few people were getting around with taped up feet now in an attempt to prevent hot spots from developing blisters or stopping already-formed blisters from getting worse. My feet were still blister free and I hoped they would stay that way.

As dawn approached, everyone finished stowing their gear

RACE DAY – STAGE 3

back into their packs and made their way down towards the riverbank. As they had done the day before, the fastest runners were wearing their shoes and socks and kept their pack strapped to their back to avoid wasting time when they exited the water on the other side of the river. Most people though, packed their backpack, shoes and socks in a dry sack and danced around from one foot to the other trying to avoid the stinging bites of the tiny ants underfoot.

Once again there was a rope strung across the river which the competitors could use to help pull themselves across, but as I found out the day before, this tended to be dragged under the water once people started to grab hold of it. I again planned to swim close enough to it such that I could grab it if I got into difficulty but would otherwise attempt to swim across under my own steam.

With a couple of support crew in the water and the drone camera buzzing overhead Shirley started her countdown from 10 to 1 in Portuguese for the start of Stage 3. As she got closer to completing the countdown more and more people joined in with the chant until it was finally time for the mad rush into the water.

The race leaders were already part way across the river by the time I gingerly walked from the ant-riddled riverbank into the muddy shallow waters and then submerged my entire body up to my neck. The warm water once again calmed my nerves and spared me the temperature shock you would normally expect when jumping into a river.

Once I was fully in the water and my dry sack was floating, I weaved my left arm through the loop made by the rolled up and buckled top of the bag and then let it trail behind me from my shoulder. I eased into a steady breaststroke, swimming parallel to, and about 5 metres away from, the guide rope.

The sun had risen over the horizon and was shining like a bright red ball in the dense air of the tropical sky. Under any other circumstances this would be a serenely beautiful moment but the thought of what lay ahead of us, and what could lie below in this water, was a definite distraction. All of my focus was on maintaining a steady pace as my arms grew weary under the strain. My strength was fading with each passing stroke and the river seemed to go on forever. People were starting to come from behind and overtake me, so I knew I was getting slower but I managed to maintain a steady stroke rate until I finally got close to the riverbank.

I maneuvered over to the rope so I could use it to help pull myself out of the water and onto the muddy riverbank. I had to feel for it under the water as it had been submerged by all the hands pulling on it. I kept testing for the bottom with my feet until I finally felt a solid base that I could use to start walking instead of swimming. It was a huge relief to give my arms a rest as I made the clumsy transition from swimming to walking.

Once I had walked far enough out of the water that my bag needed to be carried I was shocked to feel an incredible weight dragging from my shoulder. When I turned around to check on my bag I realized that it had opened up while I was in the river and was now full of water. My bag became further bloated by water as I tried to lift it out of the river. It was too heavy for me to lift so I had to drag it up onto the riverbank and then turn it around so the opening faced downhill towards the river, allowing the water to drain out of it. Fortunately most things in my backpack were packed into smaller individual dry sacks so they were protected but *unfortunately* my shoes and socks weren't among them!

Although the whole exercise of packing everything in the dry sack ended up a waste of time, I was extremely lucky that my bag hadn't actually come undone while I was in the middle of the river. Had it filled with water then, it would have sunk to the bottom of the river and probably taken me with it, or at very least leaving me with nothing and end my race. It must have come undone just as I started to pull it out of the water otherwise it would have been a dead weight on my shoulder if it had filled up while I was still swimming.

My exasperation only lasted a few moments as I quickly recovered from the mishap and re-sorted all my gear. I didn't want to waste time checking everything inside my backpack so I just recovered everything from in the outside pockets into my pack before putting on my wringing wet shoes and socks. It seems the odds were stacked against me for starting a stage with dry socks. Despite my efforts over the last two days I had still ended up with wet shoes and socks after the water crossings. I should have just kept them on my feet and saved myself the time and trouble of trying to keep them dry.

As I was preparing to head off into the jungle I saw Danielle, Ed, Karen and Jason about to leave the riverbank so I tagged along with them and hoped they would be able to help me survive the day without getting lost again. This was going to be a very long day and we would be heading deeper into the jungle as the stage progressed. I definitely didn't want to be on my own as we encroached on the jaguars home territory.

The first checkpoint was nearly 4km from the start and we travelled along undulating tracks under dense jungle canopy. The tracks were very narrow so we followed each other in single file with Ed setting the pace out front and each of us calling out warnings to others as tripping obstacles were encountered. The ground was covered with leaves, fallen logs, sapling stumps and rope-like vines. The leaves sometimes camouflaged holes formed when small tree stumps had been pulled out during the clearing of the track. These hidden holes posed the threat of twisting an ankle if you unexpectedly stepped in one and they could also be resting places for snakes that would definitely strike out at invading feet. There were plenty of spiders and furry caterpillars that clumped together to make a weird coating on the trunks of the trees, keeping our minds preoccupied and vigilant. We had so far eluded the dreaded tarantula and we hoped it would stay that way.

While making conversation, I learnt that all of them had also been attacked by the wasps the day before and it seemed everyone in the race had suffered stings except for the first few runners. While the front-runners were lucky to escape them, they must have served to stir them up and make them angry for the runners who were to follow.

With the memory of the wasp attack fresh on our minds we were hyper vigilant to anything that resembled a wasp or a bee. On a couple of occasions Jason called out "bee!!" and we all sprinted past the suspect tree with a look of absolute terror on our faces as we anticipated falling victim again to the painful stings. While we had a couple of false alarms, Danielle and I did suffer another attack,

RACE DAY – STAGE 3

which had us all sprinting off down the track until we were all clear of the threat of further stings.

I had been bitten at the base of my skull and the pain was intense for the next few minutes. At least it was only a single wasp this time instead of a hive full of them, for which I was very relieved. Once Danielle and I recovered from the pain and we all got our breath back after the crazy sprint, we once again fell into single file behind Ed and continued to follow the marker tape along the track.

Checkpoint 1 was set up along a sandy road that the race route crossed as it headed deeper into the jungle. We all stopped and rested for about 10 minutes while we filled up our water bottles and sat down to take the weight off our backs and feet.

I checked my little snacks that started the day in the outside pockets of my backpack and determined that they were unaffected by the earlier river dunking. A small plastic clip-seal bag that contained some pain killer tablets wasn't so lucky, rendering my supply of Paracetamol and salt tablets unusable. I had been taking the salt tablets as supplements but I'd have to start going without them.

Danielle was offering electrolyte tabs so I grabbed one of those and placed it in my water bladder in an effort to compensate for any salt losses I might experience. I had some of my own but they were in my medical bag at the bottom of my backpack and I didn't want to waste time or my tiny reserves of energy unpacking them and then repacking my bag.

Checkpoints 2 and 3 took us through the villages of Braganca and Marituba, which were the last two remaining indigenous communities that we would pass through.

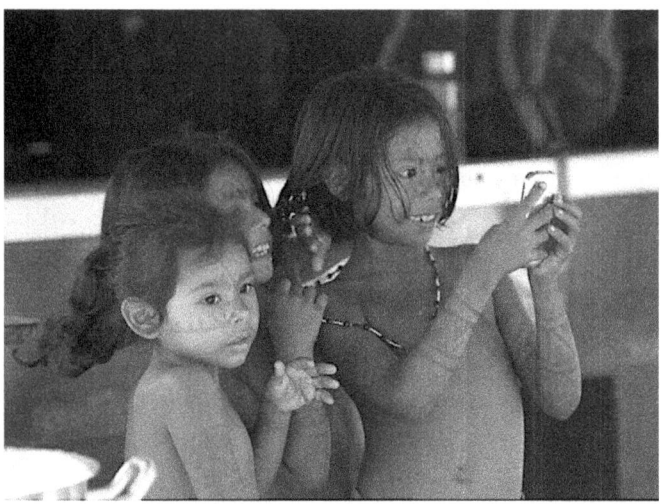

The village checkpoints generally afforded the luxury of a toilet that had thatched walls around the hole in the ground – at all the other checkpoints the jungle was your bathroom. Men definitely had the advantage over the women here as they could just turn their back and pee discreetly, whereas we poor females had to walk far enough into the jungle so we didn't shame ourselves by being spotted fumbling with damp layers of race clothes and squatting awkwardly. The thought of having a bullet ant jump up and bite me on the bum while I was relieving myself was enough to see me perform very quick toilet stops.

One of the village checkpoints had locally made handicrafts for sale and the people sported henna-like tattoos painted on their bodies. The medics and support crew got into the spirit and had similar tattoos painted on

RACE DAY – STAGE 3

their arms in playful camaraderie with the locals they spent the day with.

While resting briefly at the checkpoints I topped up my water bladder and added another electrolyte tablet to it. I was desperately craving fresh food by now so when Karen offered me some salmon jerky I thought I would give it a try. Despite not liking seafood, and never having eaten jerky before, I knew I had to try and get more food into my body so I tried just a small flake of the dried fish.

The heavily concentrated seafood taste exploded on my tongue and made me screw up my face however, within a few moments the fishy taste was replaced by a strong salty tang. Salmon jerky, along with cupuaca juice, had just become one of my new favorite foods! It was the closest thing to fresh food I was going to get for the next few days so I gladly accepted what was left in the packet when Karen offered it to me.

I was seriously doubting now whether I would have the strength to complete all 6 stages of the race. We still had the 42km of Stage 4 to do the following day and Stage 5 was meant to be 108km long, which would take all day and night to complete. That stage alone would be the equivalent of the total distance of the previous three stages combined, without the luxury of an 8 hour sleep in-between each of them! My body was totally wrecked at the end of each day after only having done 30 to 40km so I had no idea how I would be able to do two and a half times that distance in one stage. I was becoming seriously doubtful that I would survive past the first four stages.

The distance travelled from checkpoint 1 to checkpoint 3 was about 19km so we were just over half way through the stage. These two sections had many leg-crushing and soul-destroying climbs that seemed to go on forever. Shirley had warned us in the pre-race brief the night before that this stage had the longest uphill climb of the event and that when we finally thought we were at the top of it we would instead turn a bend in the track and find even more uphill struggling ahead.

She wasn't wrong! This "hill" was the Amazonian equivalent of Mt Everest, an endurance test for the hardiest of fools who dare to climb it. Most parts of it were so steep you couldn't sit down and rest even if you wanted to. It was a slow, steady slog to get to the top, with fallen tree trunks, slippery leaves, thorn-encrusted palm trees and biting jungle leaf dwellers combining to make it the obstacle course from hell.

The excitement of finally reaching the top was short-lived as what goes up must come down. The steep descent wasn't quite as bad as the ascent but it required strength and concentration to stop from sliding uncontrollably down the treacherous slope and it strained every muscle the uphill climb hadn't. Every time you grabbed a tree to control your descent you risked being bitten by ants or stabbed with 2 inch-long thorns. You had to consciously watch every single hand and foot placement to ensure you didn't either step on or grab hold of something you may have lived to regret.

As we got closer to checkpoint 4 we finally left the hills behind and continued along undulating tracks that led us even deeper into the jungle. The track was so overgrown

RACE DAY – STAGE 3

in places that it made us wonder if we were even still on the race route at times.

We were surprised to be joined by a local village man with a machete and he started making his way along the track ahead of us, clearing fallen branches and shrubs off the track with his huge knife. We were relieved each time we saw pieces of marker tape, reassuring us we were still heading in the right direction.

After struggling to navigate a particularly overgrown stretch of track, someone noticed that no marker tape could be seen in front or behind us so we stopped and evaluated our position. After a short but unsuccessful search we decided to split up, with Ed and the machete man continuing on ahead to see if they could find any signs to indicate we were still heading in the right direction, while the rest of us back-tracked towards the last piece of tape we passed. Fortunately, about 100m back we found the tiniest piece of faded tape wedged into a small notch in a tree and we figured out we had made the wrong choice at a point where the track forked.

We called out to Ed, who was still within shouting distance, and waited until he backtracked to where we were before continuing on the correct track. We were heading deep into jaguar territory and getting lost again could cost us valuable daylight and mean the difference between spending the night in the temporary base camp with armed guards watching over us or sleeping in the jaguar-dominated jungle by ourselves.

We found ourselves winding our way down into a steep gully which brought us to a small stream crossing where checkpoint 4 was set up. Although the stream wasn't very wide or deep, there had been a zip line erected for the enjoyment of the competitors. I was in agony now from the muscle pain in my upper back and neck and the last thing I felt like doing was "playing" on a zip line. After a 10 minute rest break and a couple of Paracetamol tablets from the medics, the five of us took turns at propelling ourselves along the cable to the other side of the stream. The 5-second ride was fun, but all too brief. If only that cable was 7km longer and dropped us off at the finish line!

With over 7km to go to the deep jungle camp where we would be spending the night, we knew we were racing against the clock to get there before dark. We all had a torch with us as part of our compulsory kit but navigating along these tracks, with just the tiny beam of a flashlight to guide us, would greatly increase the chances of taking a wrong turn and getting lost or of injury on the uneven ground. There was very little conversation now as we were all too physically and mentally drained to waste energy on small talk.

The only thing we could all think about was how much we were missing fresh food.

The group of four friends I was racing with had always only planned on doing the four day event so they knew that the next day would be their last stage. They were keeping their spirits up by talking about how they could eat whatever fresh village food they wanted after the end of that stage as they would no longer be required to be self-sufficient.

We were all fantasizing about how good an ice cold Coke would taste and wondering what food would be available to eat. My nutrient-deprived body was longing for

RACE DAY – STAGE 3

proper food and the more they talked about it, the harder it was for me to fight the urge to drop from the 6-stage to the 4-stage event. I was starting to accept that if there was indeed fresh food at the completion of Stage 4 then I wouldn't be able to resist the temptation. This would mean I would break the self-sufficiency rule and could no longer continue with Stages 5 and 6. With each agonizing step my resolve crumbled and I began to accept that Stage 4 would be my last day in the Jungle Marathon.

With the longest stage so far still to complete the following day, I knew I still had a long slog ahead of me to even finish the 127km event. I tried to boost my spirits with the thought that completing the 4-day event was still a respectable achievement considering I had never done a multi-stage endurance race before, but deep down I felt like a quitter. The last words my son had said to me before driving off at the airport were: "Don't quit!" and now I was seriously contemplating doing just that.

Jason was out in front and we all followed in single file. There had been many fallen tree trunks that we had to climb over but we came to one that was so huge I knew I wouldn't have the energy to haul myself and my backpack over. I took my pack off and pushed it over the top of the trunk before scrambling myself up and over, and sliding down the other side. The thought of having to put my pack on again was agonizing and I just didn't know if I had the resilience to do it.

I desperately needed a rest but didn't want to slow the others down so I told Jason to go on without me. He refused to leave me there alone and said they would all rest for a while however, I felt really bad about them losing time because of me so I mustered the energy, strapped on my pack and indicated that I was fine to keep going.

After progressing another few kilometres we came across two men who were sitting on a fallen tree across the track. One of them was clearly in a bad way and looked quite dazed with probable heat stress. The other man was keeping him company while he tried to recover enough to be able to continue. Neither of them spoke much English so it was difficult to communicate with them. Jason attempted to indicate the importance of trying to keep moving because we were getting very close to the finish line and it would be quicker to get him to the medics than waiting for the medics to come to him. After a couple of minutes he found the strength to continue and we eventually fell back into our single line formation, plodding on towards the finish line.

With less than 1km to go we came to a sudden drop leading down to a swamp. The slippery embankment was so steep it had been lined with a rope railing to hold onto while descending. Wooden planks formed a narrow bridge over the watery swamp and after crossing it we were faced with the impossibly steep climb back up the other side of the embankment. Again, there was a rope rail rigged up so you could pull yourself up the side of the hill. This would prove to be the last physically draining challenge before finally crossing the finish line in the deep jungle camp.

Deep Jungle Camp

It had been 10 hours and 50 minutes since the start of Stage 3, by far the longest and hardest race day I had ever endured. I only just made it to the finish line before the last signs of daylight disappeared. With twilight being very short-lived in the tropics, I knew it wouldn't be long before our jungle resting place was in total darkness so I wanted to find a place to hang my hammock straight away.

Unlike the previous nights, we didn't have the luxury of a spacious village camping area to spread out over. Instead, it was a very cramped clearing within otherwise extremely dense jungle vegetation. The site had been specially prepared for the Jungle Marathon and the main thing that differentiated the area from the rest of the dense jungle was that the ground had been raked clean of leaves and debris. The resulting piles of leaves now lay heaped amongst the chaotic network of gnarled tree roots that were exposed on the sandy soil.

I quickly moved away from the congested area around the finish line to make way for other competitors emerging from the jungle track behind me. At first glance the tight confined camping space already seemed to be full, so I walked around to the back of the area to try and find a couple of spare trees to hang my hammock from. I was able to find one spare tree that no-one had claimed yet but had to share the trunk of a small sapling with another competitor.

The first tree I started tying my ropes around was right

next to one of the mounds of raked leaves and I shuddered to think of what displaced ground-dwelling insects, spiders and reptiles could be seeking refuge in there. I had to stake one of my rain sheet tie-down cords into the ground right next to the mound, which would have given any unwanted little visitors a convenient route into my hammock, so I sprayed all my hammock cords with insect repellent to ward them off during the night.

I was sharing the small sapling with a competitor from the UK who had crossed the finish line two and a half hours before me, so he was already set up and relaxing after his tremendous effort. Tony, like many of the competitors, used his athletic pursuits to help raise funds for charity and his military background steered him towards a charity that helps provide for veteran servicemen and women. He had completed all three stages so far in great times despite the fact that his previous ultra-endurance experiences in desert climates were no match for this difficult jungle course.

Once my hammock was set up I changed out of my race clothes and into my camp T-shirt which, although it was getting increasingly dirty and smelly, still felt much better than the clammy clothes I had been wearing throughout the day. This camp had no river access for a swim and no shower or washing facilities so I would have to go to bed as I was. I was too exhausted to really care anyway.

Before it got completely dark I went searching for the "toilet" and was pointed to a small cleared track leading off into the jungle from the camping area. At the end of the 15m long track I found a hole in the ground with no

RACE DAY – STAGE 3

privacy screen or even trees to hide behind, just a very exposed hole in the ground. I thought "This is definitely a "men's" bathroom", so I decided to take my chances in the jungle and found a much more private area.

I returned to my hammock, grabbed one of my dehydrated meal packs and stumbled my way around the hammocks and tie-down cords over to where the race volunteers were providing boiling water. This pouch was the only remaining "gourmet" meal that I had and I was hoping the Apricot Chicken would provide the protein and carbs that my depleted body was craving. Whilst waiting the 10 minutes for the food to "cook" in the foil pouch I joined Anna, the Russian lady, on a plank of wood that had been set up as a seat.

Anna was sitting with one leg crossed over the other and seemed as fresh as a daisy. With a relaxed smile on her face and dressed in khaki Capri pants and T-shirt, she looked like she had just been for a pleasant stroll through a park rather than having just completed a grueling 3-day trek through the Amazon Jungle. She had originally signed up to just do the Stage 4 42km marathon but Shirley convinced her to give the 4-day event a go. She borrowed a suitable pack to carry all of her gear in and set off on Stage 1 with the rest of us.

While sitting there talking to Anna I tried to eat the meal I had re-hydrated but as soon as I tasted it I just knew I couldn't eat it all. It tasted like a disgusting bag of soggy chemicals and I couldn't bring myself to eat more than a few spoonfuls.

Just as I gave up trying to eat any more, Dave, the race timing official, came and sat next to me with a packet of salty crackers he was eating. The sight of "real" food made me sigh out loud and I told him how I had been craving a Coke all afternoon. Dave looked at me and excitedly said that there was Coke at the table where the water was being distributed. I looked at him in disbelief and told him to stop bullshitting me but he laughed at me and said that it was true.

Apparently all the runners were getting a cup of Coke when they finished instead of the juice that we had been given at the villages after the previous two stages. He offered to go and get me a cup of it and came back a minute later with the warmest and flattest Coke I had ever tasted however, at that moment in time it was the most unbelievably delicious drink I could think of!

I told Dave I would kill for some of his salty crackers and although he offered them to me, I agonized over accepting them because the race rules stated that we were only allowed to eat what we were carrying with us. Arghhh! I wanted those crackers so badly!! Like my body, my mind was too weak to hold out for long and I couldn't resist the temptation any longer. I gratefully accepted Dave's crackers and ate two of them straight away. I wrapped up the remaining four in their packet and took them with me as I headed back to my hammock.

I lay in my hammock to take the weight off my aching back while waiting for Shirley to begin the briefing for the following day. My neighbor, Tony, wasn't lying in his hammock but he returned soon after. When he lay down and his hammock took the full weight of his body, it caused the small tree that we shared to bow alarmingly and I suddenly found myself dropping down towards the ground. I braced as I felt it lurch down and expected to crash into the ground but fortunately it stopped short. I guess this was the jungle equivalent of sleeping in a bed with a crappy mattress and being bounced around when the person next to you moves.

My hammock was only a few steps away from Carol's and I watched as the TV Globo crew interviewed her while she lay hanging there amongst the crowded campsite. The only lights in the camp were from people's headlamps so the cameramen had set up a big floodlight to capture Carol's head as she peaked out from the security of the insect net that covered her hammock.

This campsite represented the essence of the Jungle Marathon; oppressive and gloomy jungle with absolutely no facilities or comforts. About 80 competitors and support crew were jam packed into this tiny clearing which encroached on the home turf of the freely roaming native jaguars. One of the competitors had seen a jaguar cross the track up ahead of him while running the final leg of this stage, which reinforced the need to be vigilant while roaming through, and camping in, this part of the Amazon.

Everyone was becoming more subdued in the camp during the evenings as the days wore on. The level of an individual runner's fitness not only determined the time it would take them to complete each stage but also determined how lively they would be in camp at the end of each day. Along with the medics and race volunteers, it was only the experienced ultra-endurance athletes who had enough energy at the end of each stage to participate in animated conversation. I envied their fitness and resilience and how they made it look so easy, while I was struggling to even think, let alone converse expressively with anyone.

Although Shirley still hadn't commenced the briefing for Stage 4, I just couldn't be bothered getting out of my hammock to assemble with everyone else. I had decided I would definitely be dropping back from the 6-stage event to the 4-stage event and would tell Shirley in the morning. My exhausted state compounded my disappointment at giving up on my goal of doing all six stages. I just wanted to go to sleep so I could stop thinking about how much I desperately needed fresh food and to erase the persistent upper back muscle aches from my mind.

Tony and I would spend the next 8 hours riding each others waves of restless hammock-bound tossing and turning. I fully expected that the small tree to which we were both tethered would eventually bend beyond breaking point and dump us both on the ground. However, I was happy to take my chances of such an occurrence rather than using energy I didn't have to try and find a better solution.

At first I was very self-conscious of Tony being disturbed every time I wriggled myself into a less uncomfortable position but it didn't take long for fatigue to override my concerns as I succumbed to another night of restless, broken sleep. The cooler early morning temperature again kept me from achieving a deep sleep as I woke up regularly to find myself in an uncomfortable fetal position, attempting to keep warm.

Stage 3 Race Summary

254km – Male

The first person to cross the finish line of Stage 3 was again the Austrian, Bernard, in a time of 5:11:31. Sousa (Brazil) was second, in a time of 5:27:18, followed by the third and fourth place getters who crossed the finish line almost tied with Marcelo Sinoca (Brazil) recording a time of 5:46:28 and Hiro (Japan) 5:46:29. Rodrigo Souza (Brazil) was very close behind in a time of 5:50:26.

The remaining field of competitors was well spread out, with the last to cross the finish line in a time of 12:50:03.

Brazilian Vinicius Boscolo struggled to complete the stage and made the decision not to continue with the race the next day. He would be the fifth 254km male to pull out of the race.

254km – Female

Jacqui Terto (Brazil) proved her dominance again with a convincing win in a time of 8:20:40. Marie (France) was to follow some time later with 10:09:05 and I was third over the line in this category in a time of 10:49:55.

The grueling Stage 3 course took it's toll on Kim (UK) and Jacquie Palmer (USA) with both of them crossing the line together in a time of 16:26:00, after keeping each other company while completing the final hours of the course in total darkness. What an amazing show of courage and determination by both of them to keep going and complete the stage. They would both have very little time to recover before the pre-dawn start of Stage 4.

127km – Male

Lucas Marques (Brazil) again finished first in a time of 6:22:15, which was a convincing 2 hours ahead of his closest rival. The next three people over the line all finished very close to each other with Clayton Conservani (Brazil) finishing in 8:19:03, Themos Sgouras (Greece) in 8:21:35 and Mike Kraft (Germany) in 8:23:37. The final male crossed the line in 12:51:20.

127km – Female

The first four women in this category were very evenly matched with only 12 minutes between first and fourth places. Andreia (Brazil) again showed her dominance with a time of 8:12:58, followed by Carol Barcello (Brazil) in 8:19:06 and then Stefanie Bacon (UK) in 8:19:20. These were the three fastest times for the women overall in this Stage. Danielle (USA) and Karen (Australia) would finish together in a time of 10:49:50.

Stage 3 – The Game Changer

There were more 254km competitors, besides myself, talking about dropping down to the 127km race as many others were now experiencing foot problems, body chaffing and rashes. One of the Brazilian runners had developed an inflamed big toe on his right foot, which forced him to cut off the top his shoe so he could complete the stage. Once he was back at the camp, the medics pierced his big toe nail so the blood and pus could be drained off and his scream of pain alerted everyone to the fate of yet another casualty in the hands of the medics! However, within an hour he was walking normally again and was relieved to be able to continue the race.

The ruggedness and length of Stage 3 had left everyone exhausted, a condition not helped by the confines of the deep jungle camp that we found ourselves cramped into. Everyone's spirits were definitely down and the mood was much more subdued compared to previous nights. The remaining 254km competitors weren't even half way yet and still had the daunting 108km Stage 5 to contemplate. Thinking back on how difficult the 38kms of Stage 3 had been it was hard to imagine doing 108km non-stop through similar terrain.

All of the remaining 127km male and female competitors would start the fourth and final stage of their race in the morning. Knowing that Stage 3 was supposed to be the hardest stage made it easier to prepare mentally for the challenge ahead.

Sandy, Fred and Lee re-joined us in the deep jungle camp so they could compete in the one day marathon stage race. There were some additional local competitors who joined us for Stage 4 and one of the race volunteers, Marieke, would swap sides and run Stage 4 as a competitor.

Chapter 8

RACE DAY – STAGE 4

Deep Jungle Camp to Jaguarira – 42.0km
The Marathon Stage

Stage 4 Brief

Start to Checkpoint 1: 12.27km
Checkpoint 1 to Checkpoint 2 (Pedreira): 8.80km
Checkpoint 2 to Checkpoint 3: 7.90km
Checkpoint 3 to Finish(Jaguarira): 13.03km

I could hear people moving around outside my hammock cocoon and opened my eyes to see the beams of headlamps cutting through the otherwise pitch black confines of the early morning campsite. The pre-dawn ritual had begun, as people started preparing for the start of Stage 4.

I lay in my hammock with the soft sleeping bag liner held up around my shoulders, in an effort to keep the damp coolness of the pre-dawn jungle air off my clammy skin. It wasn't really cold as such, and I'm sure most of the competitors who came from cold climates probably thought it was uncomfortably warm, but it was too cold for me. The silk liner was so light that it barely made any difference and to be honest, being entangled in it was just as frustrating as being cold. It was too hot when I'd first go to bed to be able to get into it so then I would find myself waking in the middle of the night and trying to find the opening of the long tube of material, and then having to slide my body into the slippery silk liner while laying supine and swinging in the slippery nylon hammock. It was no easy task and did my head in each and every night.

My hammock suddenly lurched down towards the ground, signally that Tony had just got up out of his hammock and that maybe it was time I should be doing the same. There was a small pocket on the inside of my hammock that I kept a bottle of water and my malaria medication tablets in which helped me stay in a routine of taking one of the tablets each morning. I awkwardly moved myself into a slightly inclined lying position so I could take a tablet with a swig of water without choking myself, and then started the ungainly maneuver of getting out of my hammock, which was made all the more difficult now that it was only inches off the ground.

I rejoiced at the thought of having survived another night in the jungle without a single ant or spider taking refuge in my hammock. Some other people had not been so lucky with one of the medics being bitten by an ant which snuck into her hammock while she was in it. I was very diligent in ensuring that my hammock was fully zipped up whether I was in it or not – I wasn't taking any chances. I was to find out later that someone had also been bitten by a scorpion while in the deep jungle camp – so glad it wasn't me!

After relieving my bladder under the cover of darkness in the jungle next to where my hammock was, I started the uncomfortable process of putting my tight, cold, damp race clothes back on. I was grateful for the pre-dawn darkness again as I pulled my T-shirt over my head and stood near-naked only metres away from other competitors who were now up and about. There were no changing rooms at this venue, that's for sure.

We wouldn't be starting with a river crossing for Stage 4 so I took delight in getting a clean pair of dry socks out of a dry sack, and pulling them on. This was the only luxury I would experience on this trip and I delighted in the fleeting moments where at least one tiny part of my body felt warm and cozy. The dry socks also helped shield me from the icky feeling of putting on wet shoes, although the dampness would eventually migrate from the shoes into the socks.

The night's sleep, as broken as it was, had re-energized my spirits to a degree and my deep disappointment in deciding to drop out of the 254km event and only do the 127km was now replaced with reserved excitement at the thought of only having one stage left to complete. Although this next stage was to be 4km longer than the previous one it was to be in slightly less challenging terrain with less of the tortuous hills, so I felt confident I could finish it.

I wandered around camp to the light of my headlamp while I prepared a small amount of macaroni cheese to eat for breakfast. Now that I was not having to make my snacks last for the extra 3 days of stages 5 and 6, it meant I no longer had to ration the few remaining packets of crisps

RACE DAY – STAGE 4

I had for any longer than today so I enjoyed the salty crispness of one of those as well. As I packed my race snacks into my backpack I delighted in knowing that I now had the remainder of the salmon jerky that Karen had given me, 4 salt crackers from Dave and two tiny snack packs of cheese rings to sustain me over the marathon stage – *what a treat!*

Because I went to bed quite early and missed the race briefing, I only found out while packing up my hammock that the people who were only doing the marathon stage, or those doing the 127km event of which Stage 4 was to be the final stage, didn't need to carry all of their camping gear with them while they were running. You only needed to carry what you would need to sustain you to the finish line.

If I hadn't already made up my mind to drop back from the 254km to the 127km then this bit of news certainly would have been the tipping point. To finally be able to lighten the load on my back was the best news I could possibly hear and immediately started offloading everything I wouldn't need and putting it into a separate bag to leave with the race organizers.

I found Shirley over in the medics area and told her I had decided to drop out of the 6 stages and just complete the 127km 4-stage event. I hated hearing myself say it out loud for the first time but the disappointment was counterbalanced by the elation of dropping my bag of surplus gear off for someone else to carry to the next campsite. I also knew this was the point of no return because completing the stage without all of my gear meant that I wouldn't have the option of changing my mind and continuing on to do Stage 5. All of the people who were still planning to do the 254km event had to still carry all of their belongings with them, so out of fairness to them we wouldn't be able to change our mind after having run one stage without it. The decision was final now.

The small campsite became a hive of activity as everyone packed up their hammocks and prepared for another day of racing. I was concerned about how long it would take me to complete the stage and if I would even be able to finish it before it got dark. The extra 4km could add an hour onto the time to take to do it if the terrain was as difficult as the previous stages had been and I definitely didn't want to still be trying to find my way through the jungle after dark.

Knowing that I found it difficult to keep up with the pace that Ed, Jason, Karen and Danielle had been setting in the final stages of the previous day I was worried that if I stayed with them again today they might be annoyed that I would slow them down. With the weight on my back much less now I knew I could probably manage to jog any flatter sections, if there were any, so I decided to make an effort to jog as much as I could from the start to try and give myself a good head start early in the day. There were a lot more people in the race today, with the extra marathon stage runners joining us, so I was hoping I wouldn't be out in the jungle by myself for much, if any, of the race.

With the first glimmer of morning twilight peeking through the jungle canopy we all began to assemble at the start banner which was set up over the narrow track that led into the jungle. I wouldn't be sad to see the back of

RACE DAY – STAGE 4

this campsite and couldn't wait to get started so we could get out of the claustrophobic jungle hideaway. I was happy to leave this place to the jaguars and get the hell out of there. After spending a night in the deep jungle I would certainly appreciate the river campsites more now.

With my brain struggling to make sense of my mixed emotions of dread, excitement and disappointment, I was left standing in a bit of a daze as I waited for the countdown to the start to begin. I really wished I had learnt to count to ten in Portuguese so I could have joined in the chant from 10 to 1 but I had to settle for counting down in English to myself instead. Because I had missed the brief the night before I had no idea what to expect in this stage but just knowing it would be my last day of racing was enough to convince myself I'd be able to get through it, no matter what the course threw at me.

The faster runners moved through the crowd of competitors to position themselves as close as possible to the start line so they didn't have to lose time trying to get past other runners once we headed into the jungle along the narrow track. It was going to be a congested start with over 60 people having to fall into a single file as soon as they crossed the start line so I moved to somewhere around the middle of the pack where I wouldn't be in the way of the faster people but would be able to start ahead of the people who I suspected would be walking instead of running. My strategy was to try and jog for as long as I could from the start, so I positioned myself accordingly.

The race began amidst excited cheers as everyone left the deep jungle camp behind. I started jogging as soon as I was free of the crowd and was amazed at how good I felt when I did. The minor decrease in the weight of my backpack made a huge difference to my agility and I found myself steadily gaining on, and then overtaking, quite a few people over the first kilometre. The crowd quickly spread out as people naturally fell into line according to their individual paces.

The track was the same as we had encountered on all the other days, complete with an anastomosing network of gnarly roots, small severed tree stumps, fallen logs, pot holes and menacing vines that doubled as trip wires. All of these threatened to trip us up if we lost concentration or diverted our attention off the track. Having to remain so alert at all times meant that it was difficult to judge time and distance, and I would lose track of both as I continued jogging at a comfortable pace.

The jungle floor here is not very densely vegetated as the overlying treetop canopy is so thick it prevents most of the daylight from penetrating it. Without direct sunlight it is difficult for smaller trees and shrubs to survive. The taller trees thrive at the expense of the smaller ones as their immense trunks shoot skywards in search of the sun.

There were many of the huge tree trunks fallen over the track that you would need to climb over. There was always a temptation to stop and rest on top of them while your straddled legs were momentarily relieved of carrying your weight, but Shirley's bullet ant bite reminded me of how dangerous sitting on a log can be out here. Being bitten by a bullet ant was a risk I wasn't prepared to take.

I was surprised to see Brazilian Jacqui up ahead of me and even more surprised to see that I was actually gaining on

RACE DAY – STAGE 4

her. When I came up behind her she pulled off the track and motioned for me to pass her but I knew there was no way I could maintain a pace that was faster than what she was capable of, so I slowed down and just stayed behind her so she didn't have to try to pass me soon after. The gap between us would eventually widen as the stage progressed but that close encounter raised my spirits and motivated me to keep jogging for as long as I could. I knew this flat ground couldn't last forever so I was keen to try and make up as much time as I could while the terrain was still manageable.

After a few kilometres of running along the narrow jungle track we came to a small stream crossing and on the other side of the stream was a cleared area with a crude shelter made from logs. There was a long wooden bench set up with some large containers of drinking water sitting on them and a couple of race volunteers offering to help people fill their water bottles. I had barely even drunk any of my water yet so I decided not to waste any time stopping there and continued to follow the marker tape that headed back into the jungle.

I had no idea how far it was to the first checkpoint but knew that at some stage we would come to a stream that we would have to swim down for over a kilometre. As the morning heated up and my clothes became drenched in sweat I longed to reach the stream so I could wash the previous 36 hours of racing sweat and stench off my body.

Everybody had spread out now and I was running by myself with no-one else in sight. The jungle track seemed to go on forever and I started cursing the whereabouts of the bloody stream. I not only desperately needed a wash but was also looking for an excuse to stop running and I didn't want to do that until I got to the stream.

I started to detect a gradual descent and was hoping it meant that I was getting closer to the stream. It quickly became steeper and I could now see a gulley starting to take shape ahead of me and soon after I was ecstatic to see the narrow track open up into a small clearing and lead onto a small log bridge that passed over a swift flowing stream.

A race volunteer was stationed at the bridge and I could see one of the competitors drifting off downstream in the strong current. Unlike the brown murky water of the rivers we had swum across, this stream was crystal clear with a beautiful sandy bottom visible.

I couldn't wait to get into the water, but stopped to put my backpack into a dry sack so I could protect it's contents from the water and also use it as a flotation device. The dry sack hadn't been used since the misadventure after the Stage 3 river crossing, where it filled up with water just as I got to the riverbank, and although I was pretty sure that was caused by the buckle coming undone, I couldn't be sure that there wasn't also a hole in it somewhere. Even the slightest hole in the sack would mean it would be useless to me for storing my bag in because if it got water inside it then it would eventually become too heavy to float.

As soon as I had everything in the dry sack I rolled up the top to lock the air in and then snapped the buckle shut to secure it. I considered my options for getting into the stream and passed up the chance to have a dramatic jump off the bridge in favor of the more reserved walking down

RACE DAY – STAGE 4

the embankment and gradually submerging myself.

The water was freezing! I was shocked at how cold it was and as the water level got further up my legs, my eager anticipation of getting into the beautiful stream quickly turned into reserved trepidation.

After hesitating for a few moments I gave in to the cold water and walked in all the way, with the water reaching up over my chest. The sudden chill took my breath away but I quickly recovered and started drifting downstream with the current. My bag was holding the trapped air for now and floated along the top of the water, providing me with a flotation device, should I need one. More importantly, however, it relieved me of the weight that I had been burdened with for the past 3 days. It felt so good to finally get the pack off my back and the weight off my legs, and let the buoyancy of the water and the power of the current propel me.

The euphoria of drifting weightlessly down the stream wore off very quickly. The first massive tree trunk that I slammed into saw to that. Within seconds of leaving the cleared area around the small bridge the stream narrowed into a deep channel with fallen trees submerged below the surface of the water which would only be detected once my shins slammed into them. I would be walking in waist deep water then without warning the bottom would disappear from under my feet and I would sink under the water and be grabbing for my sack to help keep my head above the water.

I tried to lift my knees high and lead forward with my feet to test for trees as I went but the force of the current would push my legs up against the rock-hard trunks before

I would have time to react. My skin was very cold from the frigid water, making the sudden blows to my shins and thighs all the more painful. No matter how cautious I was there seemed no way of avoiding bashing some part of your legs on the underwater logs.

There were also many large tree trunks crossed over the surface of the water that I had to try and get over which could be awkward because the deep water gave me nothing to push off from, so I had to pull my full weight up with just my arms until my belly was lying flat on the log and then swing my legs over the log and slide off the other side. I wouldn't know if the water on the other side would be deep or shallow, if I could stand on the bottom or sink underwater, so I hugged my dry sack and just keep my legs out behind me until I had a chance to feel for whether the stream was shallow enough for me to stand up and walk.

It didn't seem to matter if I was walking or floating as to whether I could avoid slamming into the submerged logs. In the shallower water my shins and thighs would bare the brunt of the blows, but in deeper water I even managed to get partly winded at one stage when I slammed into a log which was at stomach height and it knocked the wind out of my lungs.

As I progressed down the stream I was surprised to see Brazilian Jacquie again, up ahead of me. She had just come to a huge log that was fallen across the stream and I watched as she ducked under it to get to the other side. I felt anxious just watching her go under the murky water and dreaded having to do the same in a few moments.

When I got to the log I stopped to consider my options as it was so large it was going to be an effort to pull myself up and over it, but I dreaded the thought of having to go under it. There was no way to tell if there were other logs on the other side of it that could block you from safely resurfacing, and the water was quite murky and I definitely didn't want to have to open my eyes if my head was submerged. I decided to try and pull myself over it and eventually succeeded in getting past the obstacle.

Despite having the weight of my backpack off my back, and my legs not having to run for this kilometre of the route, this stream was taking it's toll on my energy. I was now cursing the bloody logs and groaned in pain with every body blow they inflicted on me. The strong current made it practically impossible to avoid being slammed into them.

As I continued downstream I saw another competitor up ahead of me and as I got closer I realized it was Alfredo, the runner I had taken a wrong turn with on Stage 1. I quickly closed the gap between us and when I did I saw that he was having trouble with his dry sack which had come undone and filled up with water. He was left with the awkward task of emptying the water out and repacking his backpack while submerged waist-deep in the fast flowing water. He had got it all under control just as I reached him so we continued down the stream together.

I went ahead and yelled out warnings every time I came to a log, trying to indicate what part of the leg it was likely to slam into so he knew to anticipate approximately what depth under the surface of the water the log was lying at. Even knowing one was coming still didn't help avoiding slamming into them a lot of the time, so we both continued the stream descent with frequent cursing and screams of pain.

Alfredo and I eventually came to the end of the stream, but the race marker tape then led us into a swamp that was like a shallow, muddy version of the stream we had just conquered. Only there were even more logs to negotiate. It looked like a log graveyard, they were everywhere! It was impossible to judge with every step what depth you would sink into the mud so you were constantly having to make corrections for the ever-changing shifting of weight as you progressed through the unpredictable swamp.

I was making frustratingly slow progress but was excited to see the race volunteers up ahead signaling that the stream and swamp legs of the race were completed and I was about to head back onto a jungle track.

The race photographer was positioned on the edge of the swamp taking photos as the competitors emerged from the shallow muddy water, and awkwardly stumbled up the embankment where there was finally firm ground under our feet. There was still no checkpoint in sight so I unpacked my backpack out of the dry sack, put it on my back and continued following the marker tape into the jungle. I had no idea how much further I had to go before reaching checkpoint 1, so just plodded along at a slow jogging pace as I kept a close eye on the race route marker tape.

The jungle canopy started to thin out and the vegetation gradually morphed into a more open expanse of sandy-soiled shrub life. The vegetation continued to show signs of a more coastal environment and the ground soon turned into loose white sand that made jogging quite difficult. There were only sparse low-lying trees and shrubs

RACE DAY – STAGE 4

now with many relics of uprooted trees lying on their sides from previous flooding events that have washed through the river basin.

The trees eventually cleared to reveal extensive white fluvial sands, indicating I was now very close to a river. Hiding under the shade of the last group of trees was Checkpoint 1.

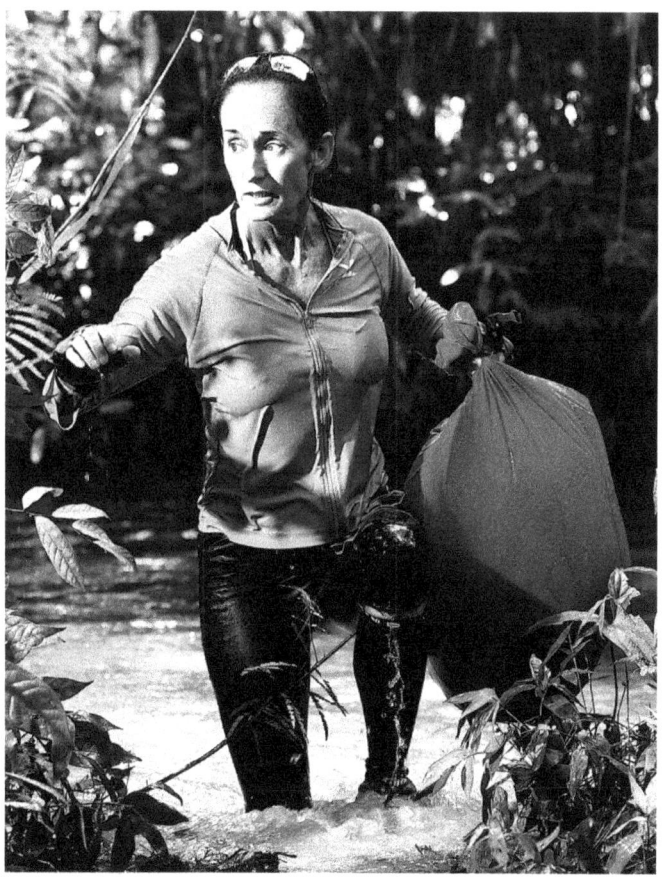

It had been over 12km since the start of the race and

the 2km of stream and swamps had slowed me down considerably. I had slowed down to a fast walk as I got closer to the checkpoint so I wasn't feeling too exhausted. My water bladder was nearly drained so I needed to fill that up, but otherwise I didn't really feel like I needed to waste much time stopping here.

My shoes had filled with sand while doing the stream section and I could feel it compacted in the space underneath my toes but it wasn't causing any discomfort so I decided to just leave it there for now. It would have taken quite a while to drag off my shoes, socks, and gaiters and put them back on again so I decided not to waste the time doing it. I would just have to put the same sandy shoes and socks back on so it hardly seemed worthwhile taking the time and effort to do it.

The checkpoint had some more of the locally made juice so I had a cup of that. It was so nice having something other than water to drink. I also enjoyed eating the remaining few pieces of the salmon jerky Karen had given me the day before and made a mental note to order some more when I got home and send it to Karen in appreciation of her generosity in my time of need!

As soon as I refilled my water bottles I was on my way again. I had only stopped for about 5 minutes but other runners were spending more time there while they took their shoes and socks off to clean the sand out of them. The longer I stayed, the harder it would have been to get moving again so I just did what I had to and then continued on.

Once I was out of the shade of the trees at the checkpoint, the sand opened out into a large white expansive sandbar that led to the riverbank. The small river was a tributary that fed into the much larger Tapajos River. Meandering channels carved through the white sand revealing relict pathways where streams had drained the jungle catchment area of the enormous amount of rain that is dumped there over the wet months.

I felt for the last bag of cheese rings that I had stored in the front pocket of my backpack and ate the several rings as I walked. The tiny pack barely satisfied me and I stopped walking while I up-ended the remaining crumbs from the bottom of the pack into my mouth. I delighted in how good they tasted and savored every last crumb.

I continued to walk over the massive expanse of sand and was grateful I had a pair of sunglasses to protect my eyes from the blinding reflection of the sun off the white sand. After spending the entire morning in the shade of the jungle canopy I was now unprotected from the hot mid-morning sun. While my long sleeves and long pants protected my skin from burning in the hot sunshine, they unfortunately kept a lot of my body heat trapped so I was hoping that I would head back into the jungle soon.

The sandbar led to a narrow, but deep, stream which we had to cross. Although it was only several metres wide, I watched as another competitor quickly dropped down to chest-deep water within a few steps of leaving the bank so I decided to put my pack into the dry sack again.

The fast-flowing stream had carved a deep meandering channel through the sandbar as it worked it's way towards the river. As my body was immersed to chest height in the chilly water I gasped out aloud and raised my arms up over my head in an attempt to spare them of the temperature shock. I went from being hot to cold in a few seconds but I knew I wouldn't stay cold for long once I was back on the track.

The race marker tape led back into a sparsely vegetated area which then came out into a large shallow water pond which was covered with tiny yellow flowers. The water was crystal clear and only a few inches deep with a base of fine white sand showing amongst the water plants and the low-lying palm trees. The sudden change in the scenery was breathtaking.

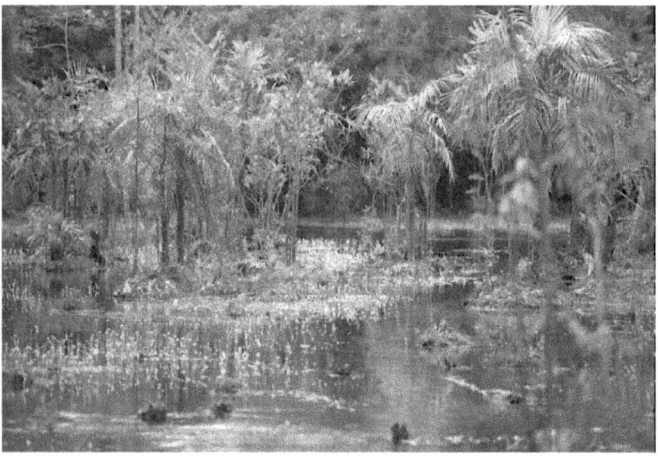

The shallow pond was about 50m across but remained only a few inches deep. It's pristine beauty was in stark contrast to the deep jungle that we had been racing through for the past three and a half days. It looked more like the Everglades than the Amazon. Tiny yellow flowers poked through the surface of the water creating a colorful blanket of foliage in the dappled sunlight.

RACE DAY – STAGE 4

The totally unexpected change in scenery diverted my attention away from my painfully fatigued body to the wonders of the Amazon that unfold as we continue in this incredible race.

Once across the pond the marker tape led back into the jungle and along more narrow trails like we had endured for most of this race. I was out on my own again now but I knew there were people fairly close by so I wasn't too concerned about venturing through the jungle by myself. I still remained vigilant though so I didn't trip over anything on the ground or miss any of the marker tape on the trees that would prevent me from getting lost.

The next checkpoint was nearly 8km from the last one and most of this distance was along jungle trails. I was entertained by the many whistling birds as I made my way along the route, and came across a few hairy spiders almost totally camouflaged by the dead leaves they were hiding in.

There were also some weird caterpillars that clumped together on the trunks of the trees and looked like a furry rug hugging the tree. These caterpillars could be seen in a lot of the places we had been running through and were always a fun distraction when I would come across another patch of them.

The trees in the jungle were generally all the same but I passed one isolated patch of giant bamboo that towered up almost as high as the jungle trees. It was an amazing sight and I regretted not having my camera with me to take a photo of it.

I eventually came out of the jungle and followed the

marker tape down a sandy road that led into a village. Children lined the road and waved with excitement as I jogged past them. I high-fived the kids along the road as their parents watched on from the front of their homes.

The sandy road came to a T-intersection with a more major road, which still had a coarse sandy surface. The marker tape led around to the right and as I turned the corner I could see another couple of competitors off in the distance. I had slowed down to a brisk walking pace now and heard someone coming up behind me. I turned around to see one of the Brazilian runners about to overtake me, and was surprised to see a huge long-bladed hunting knife strapped to one of his legs and another strapped to the front of his backpack. The Brazilians obviously took the threat of jaguars very seriously and I couldn't help but feel that I had taken my safety for granted while running around the deep jungle camp. Did this guy know something I didn't? Was the jaguar threat understated so we didn't panic? I was glad I was back in relatively civilized surroundings now so I didn't have to worry about deep jungle animals anymore…*hopefully!*

The sandy road seemed to go on forever. There were local people walking along it at times and old village vehicles driving along it. Jungle village life was going on around me as my painfully fatigued body watched from the sidelines. I felt like an out-of-place intruder in the uncomplicated lives of these people and wondered what they thought of me as I power-walked past them in my filthy race clothes and backpack.

Checkpoint 2 finally appeared ahead of me, set up in a

RACE DAY – STAGE 4

sheltered area off the side of the road. It had been very hot walking along the road in the direct heat of the midday sun and a race volunteer offered to pour cold water over my head as I walked into the shelter. It was a welcome relief and my wet layers of lycra clothing would keep me a little bit cooler now.

The Brazilian who overtook me further down the road was sitting in the shelter with his shoes and socks off and was attending to his blistered feet. My feet still felt OK but after sitting down I thought I might make use of the time to empty the sand out of my shoes, but it took me so long to do the first one that I couldn't be bothered doing the other foot so I just left all the sand in it. After filling up my water bottles I left the shade of the checkpoint and continued on my way along the dirt road.

I had only walked a short distance when the marker tape turned off the main road and headed up a sandy track along a fence line. I increased my pace a little and broke out into a slow jog and took advantage of the reasonably flat track to make up a little bit of time, as I could see up ahead of me that it would soon head uphill.

I was surprised to catch up with a couple of people who were ahead of me and we slowed down to a walk as the track started to head uphill. The hill got steeper as we got further along it and there seemed to be no end in sight to the climb. The men stopped to have a rest but I continued on and slowly plodded my heavy legs further up the steep track.

Up ahead of me I spotted the secret checkpoint that was set up to record the competitors as they passed through it, in an effort to detect if any runners cheated and took a shortcut. While walking up this hill I had noticed at least one sidetrack leading off the road that had a local guy sitting on a motorbike at the junction of the roads, and I wondered if he was there to whisk away a local runner along a short cut that would meet back up with the race route. Knowing there was such a strong history of the locals cheating in this race I couldn't help but imagine these guys sitting on their motorbike along the side of the track had ulterior motives other than just being a passive race observer.

The secret checkpoint was manned by Marcus and Mike, the two firemen from the UK. Marcus placed a tag around my wrist as proof that I had checked in and then I kept plodding up the never-ending washed-out road.

I could now see the French lady, Marie, up ahead of me and I was slowly gaining on her. I eventually caught up to her and we introduced ourselves and made light conversation with what little breath we could muster. I was longing to stop and rest but I tried to push through the urge and used Marie as a pace setter.

It was hard to imagine that this road was still used by vehicles as it was extremely washed out with deep gullies running down the length of it, winding their way from one side to the other. The wet season had taken a toll on the sandy surface and the steepness would have compounded the effects of fast-flowing streams of run-off that torrential tropical downpours produce.

Finally the steepness of the track started to ease off and my body had a chance to recover from the effects of the exertion. It's incredible how a change in incline can have such a dramatic effect on your legs and heart. The screaming burn in my legs gradually eased off and Marie and I rejoiced when we finally got to flatter ground.

The track we were on eventually brought us out onto a bigger road onto which we took a left turn and then followed the marker tape hanging from the overhanging tree branches.

The road had a well maintained sandy surface and was used to access all the local villages. We were out in the full sun now and it was very hot walking with all of our gear. I had no idea what route conditions still lay ahead of us and whether we would re-enter the jungle or have more hills to conquer. I dreaded the thought of having to scramble up any more jungle hills like those that we faced in Stages 1 and 3, and was happy to stay on the relatively flat road and put up with the hot sunny conditions.

We finally spotted checkpoint 3 up ahead and gave the medics an exhausted forced smile when we walked off the road and into the shaded area that had been set up. I headed straight for the blue tarpaulin that had been laid out on the ground and took my backpack off so I could stretch out on my back. Getting the weight off my back and legs was a welcome relief but I knew it would be short-lived. I ate the remaining two salt crackers I had and washed them down with the warm water from my water bottle.

I asked one of the medics how far it was to the next checkpoint and she replied that this was the last checkpoint before the finish line but unfortunately we still had over 13km to travel to get there. This was the furthest distance between any two checkpoints that we had to cover for the entire 4 days of this event so it was bittersweet news to hear. I just hoped there were no more energy-sapping hills or swamps in those last 13km because my body and mind were too exhausted to deal with them. Despite the extreme heat on the open road I still preferred that to the extreme terrain under the jungle canopy.

After resting for about 10 minutes I filled my water bottles and then Marie and I geared up for our final leg of the day. We thanked the volunteer crew and bid farewell as we left the shade of the roadside stop and continued along the sandy road in the heat of the mid-afternoon sun.

The road was undulating with alternating long uphill and downhill sections so we decided to jog the downhill and walk the uphill in an attempt to cover the 13km as quickly as we could. The effort required to break into a jog was a huge strain on our extremely fatigued bodies but once we got going, the momentum from the gravity-assisted downhill motion helped maintain a slow but steady speed. As soon as the road started to head uphill again it was like hitting a brick wall, with momentum having to be generated by our legs, not gravity.

As we alternated between jogging and power walking we overtook two local Brazilian competitors who were walking at a fairly slow pace. They seemed to be maintaining their pace and talking to each other so we just gave them a wave and kept going. I would later find out that they would struggle to finish and became considerably affected by the heat and humidity.

The further we continued down the sandy road the less likely it was that we would have to go back into the jungle and suffer through any more of the agonizingly steep hills. With every kilometre that passed I felt more confident that

RACE DAY – STAGE 4

the hardest part of the race was behind us. I started to feel quietly excited about closing in on the finish line and daydreamed about celebrating with a cold bottle of Coca-Cola. I was so close to finally eating fresh food for the first time in nearly a week and I started thinking about all of my favorite foods and how I would never take them for granted again - how special a boiled egg will be the next time I would get to eat one!

A race support motorcycle with a bottle of water strapped to the back of it came passed us and Marie flagged it down to try and get some water to top up her water bottle, but the rider told us there was a water stop just up ahead so we signaled that we would stop there and he continued on his way. I was struggling to maintain even a power walk now and Marie jogged ahead of me in an attempt to stop at the water station and refill her bottles and then have me catch up to her, but she never stopped and I didn't see a drink stop anywhere so she must have just kept running until she got to the finish line.

I just kept walking and soon noticed that the road took a turn to the right and was now running parallel to a river that was only about 20m off to my left. As I looked ahead I could see something strange on the side of the road and as I got closer I could make out something black and white that looked like a big cow. I was focusing all of my concentration on it as I continued to walk towards it, trying to figure out what the heck it was and finally got close enough to realize that it was Yoshi dressed in his cow suit.

He was waving at me and urging me on and clapping enthusiastically. I couldn't believe it and broke into a broad smile at the sight of him and cheered back in appreciation.

He was indeed a gentle giant with a heart of gold. He must have been sweltering in the heavy suit but he was there to encourage the exhausted runners as they approached the finish line.

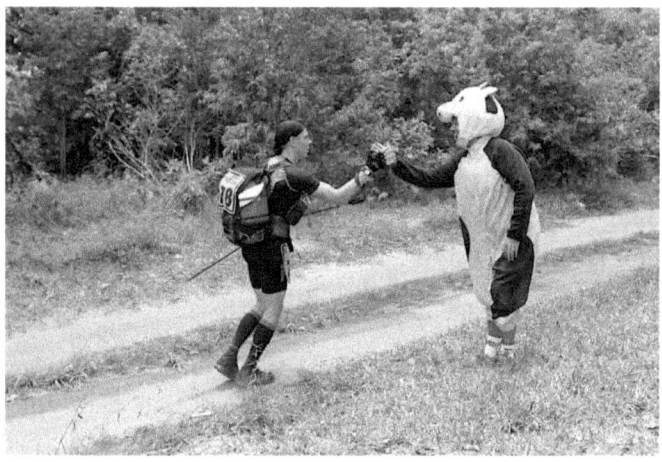

A little further on I could see some local people along the side of the road up ahead and when I got to them I saw the race directors riverboat moored at the riverbank next to a clearing where the people were. They were preparing a meal at a large wooden table in the clearing by the riverbank and I excitedly hoped that it was being cooked for us. I could smell the finish line now and felt that I was surely only minutes from finishing the race.

I couldn't wipe the smile off my face as I saw race people standing around up ahead – surely this must be the finish line! I followed the crowd and veered to the right that led into a track that led down to the riverbank and finally I could see the finish line banner. I pulled my Australian flag out of the pocket in my backpack and held it over my head as I jogged under the banner and over the imaginary finish line. Finally it was over!

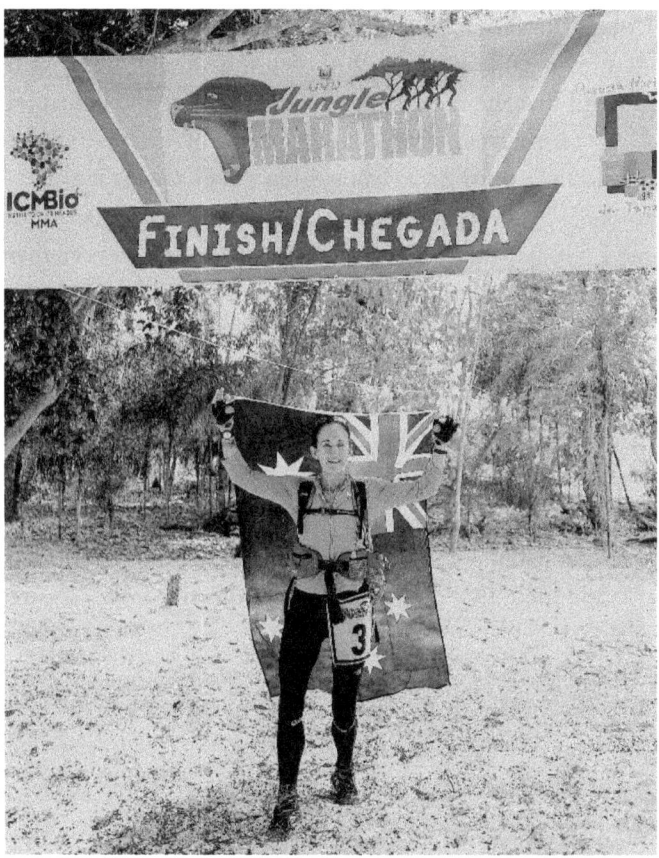

Alex, the race photographer, was there taking my photo as I finished and much to my utter amazement Dave, the race time-keeper, came up and congratulated me with a bottle of Coke! It was the greatest reward I could possibly have hoped for. Nothing has ever tasted as good as that Coke did and surely there would be no better advertisement for the beverage than having someone race through Amazonian swamps, fast-flowing streams, jaguar-infested jungle and steep never-ending hills just to get a drink of Coke! It would put the old "Solo" drink ad to shame.

My exhausted body and delirious mind were both grateful that the race was now over. Despite my jubilation, I was conscious of an undercurrent of disappointment within me at not completing what I had originally set out to do. With everyone around the finish line congratulating me I felt like a bit of a fraud and that I didn't deserve their adulation considering I was now officially a drop-out.

I knew I was being hard on myself but that didn't stop me from feeling like a quitter. The best I could do was reassure myself of the fact that I had just completed four days of the toughest race I had ever competed in and it was still far beyond any challenge I had completed in the past. To be honest though, at this point in time I think I was probably more relieved it was now over than disappointed that I had dropped down to the shorter event.

Without wasting any more time I went looking for a place to hang my hammock so I wasn't fighting for trees with the runners who were to finish behind me. There were still about 27 runners yet to complete Stage 4. It was always a dreaded part of each day, trying to find suitable trees to tie up to when you were physically exhausted. Once you got that over with though, you could relax for the rest of the evening.

The campsite was set up on the sandy banks of a tributary of the Tapajos River with the mouth of a jungle stream forming a wide delta of sand fanning out as it converged

RACE DAY – STAGE 4

with the brown waters of the river.

The clear-watered effluent from the stream trickled over the white sands of it's deltaic mouth forming deep ripple marks in the sand and creating a beautiful water feature that looked like it belonged on a tropical island rather than deep in the Amazon Jungle.

All of the trees closest to the medics area and the finish line were taken so I walked further down the sandy bank towards the river until I could find a spare tree to hang my hammock from. I found a spot where some of the Brazilians were camped and shared a tree with two of them. A gnarly old fallen log lay in the sand next to my hammock and I used it as an anchor for the ties of my rain sheet.

Once my hammock was sorted I was desperate to get my race clothes off as I had developed chaffed areas throughout todays stage and was anxious to remove the clothing that was causing the uncomfortable rubbing. In the latter part of the day I started to feel a sting where the edge of my knickers rubbed against the top inside of my legs. I found myself pulling at my knickers as I was walking in an attempt to prevent the rubbing, but there was little I could do to stop it. I also became aware of my backpack rubbing on the lower part of my back so I suspected there could have been a rash there too by now.

I grabbed my bikinis out of my bag and went to the toilet to change. We had the luxury of four different holes in the ground to choose from at this campsite and they each had three thatched walls around the hole with the fourth side open to the jungle. It doesn't get any better than this I thought to myself!

When I pulled my tights off I was surprised to see a

line of water-filled blisters along the pants line on both of my legs. The blisters were raised about 5mm up off the skin around my crotch line and looked really nasty. I was so glad I didn't know they were there while I was still in the race because I would have been mortified. I was only expecting a bit of chaffing rash, not full-blown blisters.

When I pulled my shirt off I craned my neck to see behind me on my lower back and could see raw patches of skin just above my hip bones. My backpack had slowly been wearing away at my skin as I jogged and left me with two angry red patches on my lower back. They would be fine once the air got to them and dried out, but I wasn't sure what to do about the blisters along my crotch line. I cringed at the thought of going to the very public medics area and spreading my legs for them to check out the damage I had done, so reconsidered my options. I convinced myself it really wasn't that bad – even though it looked ghastly and stung like hell – and decided to just let it air out and hope it wouldn't get infected in the meantime. I put my bikini on and made my way down towards the river.

The crystal clear stream water looked very inviting so I started walking through a narrow channel that it was flowing through where it merged with the brown river water and made my way over to a sandbar that had formed on the other side of it.

I was surprised to feel that the water was very cold and as it got further up my legs I began to rethink my plan of submerging my whole body in it.

Marie was already sitting on the sandbar with her legs outstretched in the water while she talked to another competitor, Marcelo. I went and joined them and sat next to her with my legs and bottom submerged under the freezing water, but found that the water caused a biting sting on the blisters along my crotch line and chaffing on my lower back, which made it very uncomfortable to stay there.

I desperately wanted to submerge my whole body under the clear water but it was too cold and I couldn't bring myself to do it, so I just splashed it up over myself with my hands and gave myself a mini wash instead. I was later to find out that the browner river water it merged with was a much friendlier tepid temperature and I would soak my body in that for a much needed bath.

While sitting next to Marie and Marcelo I overheard them talking about someone being disqualified, but didn't know who they were talking about and didn't like to sound nosey by asking them for more details so I just kept to myself. The stinging in my crotch and the unbearable ache in my upper back and neck made it too uncomfortable to stay sitting there propped up on my arms with nothing to take the weight off my back so I decided to head back to the camping area.

I couldn't see Karen, Danielle, Jason or Ed anywhere so went over to the finish line to ask Dave if they had finished yet. He said they hadn't, so I thought I would wait there to congratulate them when they came over the line.

While waiting, I could see some people drinking from coconuts that a village lady was slicing the top off with a huge machete. I asked someone about it and they said that this was our complimentary fruit juice for this stage of the race and all the runners were allowed to have one.

I approached the lady who was sitting cross-legged on the ground surrounded by coconuts and indicated I wanted one. She sliced a small opening into the top of a coconut with a few swipes of her machete and handed it to me. I up-ended the coconut over my mouth and devoured the sweet water that poured out of it. I was surprised how much it contained, and it took me several swigs to drain it dry. There must have been about 600ml of the milky juice inside it and I finished every drop.

I noticed someone ask the lady to cut his empty coconut in half and then proceed to eat the white internal flesh of the coconut with a spoon. With my body craving fresh food I raced to do the same and grabbed a spoon out of my pack and began to scrape the layer of white coconut from the hard husk of the shell.

I was surprised to see that the flesh came away from the husk relatively easily as it was quite soft and had a rubbery texture, rather than the hard, thick, white flesh I was used to seeing in coconuts. It was also very soft and juicy, rather than dry and fibrous like you would expect. It was the most exquisite thing I had tasted in the past 6 days and I didn't stop until the coconut shell was cleaned out of it's juicy white flesh. Mother Nature was certainly doing a good job of re-calibrating my "things to be grateful for" scale on this trip!

With the last of the daylight fading quickly, I spotted Ed and Danielle marching valiantly towards the finish line, their smiles broadening as they closed in on it. I could sense my body mimic the sense of elation they would have been feeling, knowing exactly how relieved they would have felt, having done the same thing myself just a short time before. About five minutes later Karen and Jason joined them at the finish line. In a true spirit of camaraderie the four of them had stuck together throughout the entire four stages, encouraging not only themselves, but also me for two of those days.

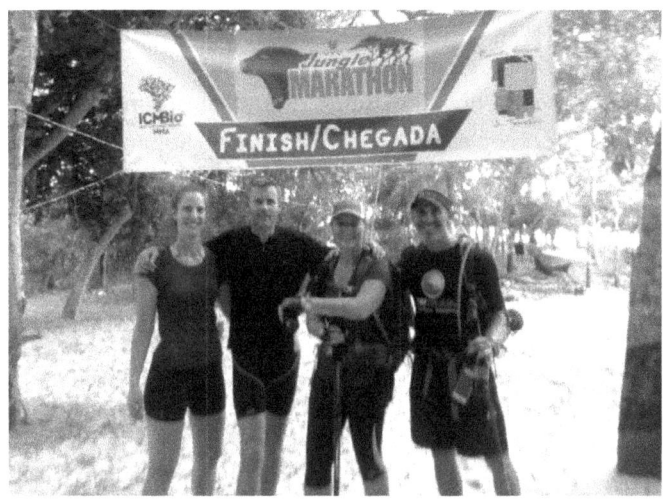

It was disappointing to see that the race photographer seemed to have knocked off for the day and their triumphant finish was void of the fanfare that earlier finishers had enjoyed. I wanted to take a photo of them crossing the finish line but I still hadn't collected my camera from Shirley from when I had given it to her at the end of Stage 1. They all had cameras with them so they took photos of each other posing under the finish line banner. It was a very understated finish to a truly remarkable achievement.

Dave came to the rescue again and surprised them all with a bottle of coke and they appreciated the gesture just as I had earlier.

I went looking for Shirley to see if I could collect my personal belongings that I had culled out of my race pack at the end of Stage 1, and then see if there was anywhere I could buy some food. My bag was stored on the riverboat that I had seen where the village people were cooking food just a few hundred metres up the track.

After collecting my things I mulled around the area where the people were cooking, in the hope that it was being prepared for the Jungle Marathon people but it soon became obvious that it was just their normal, every day family dinner. No guests invited. I was once again faced with the prospect of suffering through yet another meal of dehydrated food. That elusive meal was getting closer but still not quite there yet!

I had earlier asked Dave where he got the Cokes from and he said there was a brick hut across the road from where the riverboat was, so I decided to check it out and see if I could buy another coke and if possible, some food.

There was an old lady inside the brick shelter and I asked her if she had any Coke, but she couldn't understand any English so I repeated the words "Coca-Cola" and motioned with my arms and head as if I was drinking from a bottle. Her face lit up in acknowledgment of what I was asking and she led me to another crude building about 15m behind the one we were at and went inside and brought out a 1 litre bottle of some sort of cola. When I asked if she had "Coke" she shook her head and gestured that this cola was all she had. It was better than nothing so I asked her if I could have two of them and she grabbed another one for me. I had no idea of what a fair value was

RACE DAY – STAGE 4

for a bottle of cola in these parts but I would have paid almost anything for it at this point in time, so I handed her some Real notes and she seemed to be happy so I thanked her and left.

The drink was warm but I still enjoyed the fizzy sweet taste as I skulled from the bottle. I was so sick of drinking water and electrolytes that anything else was a welcome change. When I got back to the camp I offered the second bottle to Ed for the four of them to share in case the "shop" was to run out of stock later on.

While walking back towards my hammock I noticed one of the male competitors sitting on the ground next to his hammock with his legs spread out as he applied cream to a line of blisters along each side of his crotch – just like mine!! I had a giggle to myself as I thought how easy it is for a guy to do something like that, but it would be quite inappropriate for a female to be seen in that same position. I was at least glad that I wasn't the only person with nappy rash!

There were quite a few people having their feet attended to by the medics and I was quietly grateful at completing another endurance event without suffering a single blister, bloody toenail or chaffing on my feet. It seems my feet are truly made for running!

The only visible sign of injury I had was a bruise above my right knee that I got from slamming into the submerged logs during the stream descent. Fortunately my long tights prevented me from suffering any open wounds and I saw lots of men who weren't so lucky. Carol, the TV Globo journalist, was sporting a huge bruise that covered half of her left thigh, and it was likely to look even worse over the next couple of days.

At about 8pm we all assembled next to the finish line while Shirley gave a brief for Stage 5. This is the "long" stage and the 108km will take all day, and possibly all night, to complete. The start time would be 4:30am to give everyone the best chance of completing as much of the distance as possible in the daylight.

At the time of giving the brief, there were still five people who had not yet completed Stage 4 and were having to finish in the dark. Two of these people, Jacquie and Kim, would be continuing on with Stage 5, so they would get very little rest between finishing Stage 4 and starting Stage 5 which would mean they would be on their feet for much of the two days and two nights – a daunting prospect.

Once the briefing was over I went back to my hammock and was relieved to finally being able to rest my legs and back. I couldn't wait to lie down and get the weight off them and try to get some sleep so my body could start to recover from the punishment it had been subjected to in Stage 4.

I would have loved to have been up for the start of Stage 5 to give moral support to the ultra-endurance diehards who were still in the race, but I didn't know if I would be able to wake up for it. I hoped the movement of people preparing for it might wake me but I also sort of hoped I could just keep sleeping. I zipped myself into my suffocating cocoon of a hammock and planned to sleep, or stay lying down, until I had a reason to do otherwise.

RACE DAY – STAGE 4

My hammock was collecting more and more sand in the bottom of it as the days passed and the silk liner was getting horribly smelly, as was my T-shirt. How I longed for a shower, clean clothes and a comfortable bed at the end of the day.

I'd only been able to get broken sleep every night but I knew that even lying down for several hours was giving my body the rest and repair time it desperately needed, regardless of whether I was asleep or not. As the days wore on I was getting more sleep each night as the cumulative fatigue after four days of racing wore down my body.

After wriggling around to find a comfortable position in the banana-shaped cocoon I closed my eyes and mentally blocked out the gritty sand that was sitting between my skin and the nylon hammock and welcomed the soothing relief that my relaxed body was now feeling. I couldn't help but think of the people who were still out on the track, in the dark, yet to finish Stage 4 and was so glad I wasn't one of them. I felt guilty going to bed before they even got back and wished I was strong enough to be there to congratulate them when they crossed the finish line, but obviously their resolve was much stronger than mine. They were the true ultra-endurance athletes - I was a "wanna-be" one who had finally found her limits.

As I lay there, drifting closer to the point of unconsciousness, all I could dwell on now was that point in time when my conscious mind would finally succumb to sleep and the gritty sand, aching back, smelly clothes and claustrophobic hot hammock would all disappear. What a fantastic elixir sleep is – it can eliminate your entire existence in the proverbial "bat of an eyelid" and that's exactly what I was looking forward to now. Tomorrow would be another day and I'd worry about it when it arrived.

Emergency Assembly of Competitors and Crew

My blissful "state of being" was abruptly interrupted as I was woken by someone poking at me through my hammock. As I struggled to come back to the "real world" my brain frantically tried to make sense of what was happening and it took several seconds to register the calls from people outside informing everyone that Shirley had called an emergency meeting.

I reactively tried to hurry out of my hammock but soon realized that hammocks aren't compatible with fast movements and I risked tumbling out onto the ground with my legs entangled in the nylon web. I quickly recovered and reverted back to my usual slow and controlled method of alighting from my hammock, grabbing my headlamp and securing it to my forehead as I sat up.

A check of my watch showed that it was after 11pm which sent my mind racing with thoughts on what could possibly have prompted such a late meeting. The fact that the people who were continuing on with Stage 5 would be having a 4:30am start made it all the more bewildering because they desperately needed all the sleep they could get, so a decision to deprive them of that wouldn't have been made lightly.

Everyone staggered in confused silence, trying to negotiate the tangled web of hammock tie down cords that crisscrossed erratically throughout the dark campsite. Most people would already have been asleep when the meeting was unexpectedly called so were groggy and still trying to wake up properly as they made their way to the assembly area near where the finish line had been.

As I watched the crowd gathering in front of where Shirley was standing, I wondered if everyone else was completely in the dark about what was going on as what I was. My mind was grappling to even come up with a theory about what the race director was about to speak to us about, but I just hoped that all the competitors who were still out in the jungle when I went to bed got to the finish line safely and no-one had seriously hurt themselves…*or worse.*

Most people turned their headlamps off now so they weren't shining in peoples eyes, as we congregated in a semicircle around Shirley. I couldn't help but draw an analogy to a tribal council on an episode of "Survivor" and had a little chuckle to myself as I wondered if one of us was going to be "eliminated" and sent home. With the TV Globo cameraman filming the unfolding scene it definitely had a reality TV feel about it but unfortunately this was very real and I knew something must have been terribly wrong to have us all standing here in the middle of the night.

Once the movement had quieted down and it looked like everyone was present, Shirley began to explain the extraordinary sequence of events that had unfolded earlier in the day that I had no idea of even happening.

While it was news to me, many had already known that the runner who was first to cross the finish line of Stage 4 had been spotted riding on the back of a motorbike throughout the latter stages of the race, and when Shirley had been notified of this she disqualified the him.

With her saying this I quickly recalled the conversation I had overheard while sitting on the riverbank and realized this must have been what they were talking about.

The Brazilian runner lived in a community that Stage 5 of the race would see runners passing through. The person went back to his village after being told he was disqualified but later returned to our camp, along with members of his family, and threatened Shirley, the race director, and all the runners who were to pass through their community the next day, with harming them.

As soon as she explained the situation I automatically recalled the incident I had read in the news before coming to Brazil about the football referee who had been stoned to death then decapitated after he had fatally stabbed a player when he refused to leave the field. I was now camped in the Amazon Jungle in the very same part of the world where that savage attack occurred only a few months before. These people clearly don't live by the same rules as we do. Their uncivilized ancestry and centuries of political and religious unrest has resulted in a very different set of values towards human life than what many of us outsiders live by.

I was sure Shirley would also understand the unpredictable nature of the local people and realize that she could ill afford to pass this off as an idle threat. Although the runners agree to compete at their own risk in adventure events such as the Jungle Marathon, Shirley is still morally, and legally, obligated to ensure their safety to the best of her ability. This situation now posed a very serious dilemma for Shirley – one that had taken her until

RACE DAY – STAGE 4

11pm at night to decide what course of action she would take.

Knowing that so many people had put a considerable amount of time, money and training into coming to this event she knew how disappointed they would be if the final two stages were cancelled. Despite the threats to shoot her, Shirley made the decision to continue the race but to re-route it so the runners didn't have to travel through the disqualified persons community.

Because of the incredible logistical task she now faced, Shirley knew the start time would have to be changed from the original time of 4:30am as she would now be spending all night and tomorrow morning designing and organizing the new route. She announced a new start time of 10am so everyone knew they could sleep in and recover for as long as possible before starting the 108km stage.

This must have been music to Kim and Jacquie's ears as they had not long crossed the finish line for Stage 4, along with a few other competitors, but they were the only ones to be continuing on to Stage 5. They would now have a few more hours to rest and recover before heading off again.

I got the impression many of the Brazilians thought Shirley was overreacting to the threat, and I even overheard one of them commenting on the validity of the cheating allegation itself, but I was not doubting anything Shirley had said and I sympathized with her on the predicament she was now facing. (I was to find out later that Shirley was actually one of the people who saw the runner on the back of the motorbike).

It would be a long night for Shirley, Vicky (the

paramedic), and John Vonhof (the foot guy), as they stayed up and worked together to re-route the course. Divided loyalties and confusion would reign in the 24 hours ahead and the cultural divide had now tainted the experience for everyone.

I wanted to stay up and try to find out more about what had happened when the disqualified runner had come back and made the threats, but I was too tired and decided to go back to my hammock and leave the gossip-seeking mission until the next morning. The thought of marauding natives attacking the camp as we slept did cross my mind but I was too tired to dwell on it and just hoped my imagination exceeded the reality of the situation. It didn't stop me from getting back to sleep and I was happy knowing that I would see the start of Stage 5 after all.

Stage 4 Race Summary

254km – Male

After the disqualification of the Brazilian, the first place went to Bernard (Austria) in a time of 4:46:06, proving his dominance after now crossing the finish line first in every stage. Marcelo Sinoco (Brazil) followed in a time of 5:10:33 and third over the line in a time of 5:47:16 was Rodrigo Souza (Brazil). Hiro, (Japan) who had been in a top three placing on all the previous stages, was unfortunately affected by the heat and humidity and struggled to maintain his form. Finishing in a time of 7:59:29 would mark an end to his Jungle Marathon challenge.

The remaining male runners were well spaced out with

the final competitor crossing the finish line in a time of 10:46:11.

After completing Stage 4 there would be five runners drop out and not continue on to the start of Stage 5.

254km – Female

Jacqui Terto (Brazil) was a clear winner out of the 254km women, finishing in a time of 8:00:10. Marie was second in a time of 8:47:27 and I crossed the line soon after in 8:49:24. Kim and Jacquie (US) showed their tenacity over the difficult 42km route by continuing on after dark and arriving at the finish line well into the late evening in times of 13:38:09 and 14:03:55 respectively.

Brazilian Jacqui, Marie, Kim and US Jacquie were all still in the race and resting up for the start of Stage 5. I was the only female in the 254km category who would not go on to start Stage 5. The fact that I had dropped my bag weight for the running of Stage 4 meant that I would not qualify to line up for the final two stages even if I had wanted to now.

127km – Male

Lucas (Brazil) was a clear winner in the 127km category in 5:55:04. It would be nearly two hours before Mike Kraft (Germany) would cross the line in second place with a time of 7:35:42, soon followed by Themos (Greece) in 7:45:57. The rest of the field were staggered in their times with the final competitor crossing the finish line in

10:29:46.

Of the ten people registered to do the 127km event there was only one who failed to complete all four stages.

127km – Female

Andreia Henssler (Brazil) and Stefanie Bacon (UK) crossed the line together with a time of 6:43:20, which was well ahead of the rest of the field. Carol Barcello came in third in a time of 8:10:26

All of the competitors in this category completed the full four stages.

42km – Male

For the first time this year the Jungle Marathon included a stand-alone 42km marathon distance stage. The international competitors travelled with the group from day 1 while the local competitors joined the group in the deep jungle camp where the stage started from.

First over the finish line was Orlando de Sousa Patrocinio (Brazil) in a remarkable time of 4:52:56, followed by Leandro Ribeiro Vas (Brazil) in a time of 5:20:24 and Marcelo Alves (Brazil) in third place with a time of 5:30:37.

42km – Female

There were only two women in this category, with Alaene Xavier dos Santos (Brazil) finishing first in a time of

RACE DAY – STAGE 4

8:37:16 and Sandra Simons completing the stage in a time of 14:22:02.

Chapter 9

RACE DAY – STAGE 5

Jaguarira to Pajucara – Approximately 108 km

Stage 5 Brief

Start to Checkpoint 1: 10.5km
Checkpoint 1 to Checkpoint 2: 9.5km
Checkpoint 2 to Checkpoint 3: 9.1km
Checkpoint 3 to Checkpoint 4: 19.0km
Checkpoint 4 to Checkpoint 5: 9.3km DARK ZONE – you must arrive before 14:30 hrs
Checkpoint 5 to Checkpoint 6: 15.0km
Checkpoint 6 to Checkpoint 7: 8.1km
Checkpoint 7 to Checkpoint 8: 6.7km
Checkpoint 8 to Checkpoint 9: 8.0km
Checkpoint 9 to Checkpoint 10: 8.3km
Checkpoint 10 to Finish: 4.6km

Waiting For Stage 5 to Begin

As I lay in my hammock, I could hear the camp coming to life outside. It was broad daylight, and it felt great not having to be up and preparing my race gear for another grueling day in the jungle. I was hoping the fact that I

RACE DAY – STAGE 5

hadn't been woken up again throughout the night meant there were no added dramas to what the race director already had when I went to sleep last night, and the rescheduling of the start of Stage 5 was going ahead successfully.

After climbing out of my hammock, I navigated my way to the toilets through the maze of hammocks, stepping over some of the tie down cords and ducking under others. Most people were up and about already but were at a loose end as to what to do, now that the start time was much later than planned.

Once I was in the relative privacy of the hole-in-the-ground toilet, I checked to see what the blisters around the pants line in my crotch looked like. I was surprised to see that the blisters were no longer there and the fluid had been re-absorbed into my body, leaving just a hint of wrinkled skin that had already started to harden into a soft scab. The decision to avoid putting any cream on it and just let it dry out had paid off and the body's natural healing process was taking over like a charm.

I turned to see the worn patches on my lower back and they had done the same. The red, raw skin that was there last night had now darkened into a soft scab that would eventually harden up and protect the underlying nerve-filled layers of skin from being aggravated. They no longer stung when touched and I marveled at how efficiently the human body can repair itself. The quicker the scab can form, the quicker the infection-prone raw flesh underneath it can be protected from the elements. No amount of pharmaceutical intervention works better than "the scab".

I had no idea what the plan would be from here on for

those who weren't continuing in the race, and the thought of having to spend another two days and nights in jungle camps was daunting. Shirley was nowhere to be seen and no-one really seemed to know what was going on in respect to race changes.

I joined some of the other runners who had finished their last stage of the race the previous day as well, in the hope they would have a bit more information about the plan moving forward. With Shirley being the only English-speaking member of the organizing group, there was really little we could do but wait for her to make an announcement. We all discussed the possibility of somehow getting transported to Santarem, which is where the race was planned to finish, and wait in a hotel for the next two days. As soon as we started talking about the possibility of getting out of the jungle camp and into a comfortable hotel, I started to get excited.

Although I felt guilty about wanting to leave the main group before the final stage of the race, the thought of getting to sleep in a real bed and eat real, fresh food was overwhelming. With so much confusion in the camp at the moment, I suspected Shirley would be happy to have less people to have to try and organize. The problem we faced though, was that we couldn't just jump on a passing bus or call a taxi – we were still in the middle of the jungle! Having to transport people to Santarem after Stage 4 was not part of the original plan.

With the retribution aimed not only at Shirley but also at the runner who was currently leading the race, Bernard made the decision not to continue. He pulled out of the race and would not be starting Stage 5, and wished to go back to Santarem and then fly back to Austria. This revelation rocked the camp and Bernard distanced himself from everyone by seeking refuge on the riverboat that the film crew were camped on. There seemed to be a minority sentiment that Bernard was in some way responsible for all that was happening, which I just couldn't quite make sense of. In any case, it appeared Bernard feared for his safety should he remain.

The race timekeeper also chose to leave, stating that he wanted to make sure Bernard got to Santarem safely, but I'm guessing he was more than a little bit concerned about his own safety as well. This left the race organizers with no timing facility at all and with a huge amount to deal with already it would just add to the chaos.

Everybody's loyalties were now being tested. Without even seeing Shirley, I sensed that she must have been feeling very much on her own in trying to find a solution that would keep everyone happy. She had been up all night trying to re-route the course to make it safe for the competitors who would be continuing with Stage 5 and 6, but her Brazilian group of supporters were clearly not giving her much assistance. It was obvious they didn't share her concern about the threat and thought she was over-reacting to the situation, so were reluctant to literally lose any sleep over it themselves. As a result, it ended up being Shirley, Vicki and John who had to plan it all.

When I finally found Shirley, I asked her if it was possible to spend the next couple of days in Santarem and she said she was trying to organize transportation for all the people who wished to do the same. I had no idea how she would do it but left it in her capable, and extremely tired, hands.

As the morning progressed it became clear the race would not be starting at 10am. Shirley called a meeting to tell everyone that the start time was now going to be 2pm, in order to give the race support crew time to re-mark the race route and position medics and volunteers at checkpoints.

The mood amongst the assembled group of people was subdued. Instead of the carefree jovial banter of previous race briefings, there were now divided groups, all with different agendas.

Shirley looked exhausted, and you could sense how devastated she must have been feeling as her 12 months of planning and preparation was unraveling around her. Changing the course was still not a guarantee there would be no trouble from the restless natives. The possibility of someone getting hurt would have been weighing very heavily on her mind, and she could live to regret the decision to continue on with the race, instead of cancelling it.

I was glad not to be in her shoes and having to be responsible for what would happen over the next few days. Given the turn of events, I just wanted to get out of there.

There were now several people wanting to go to Santarem so Shirley was trying to organize how to get us all there. It was impossible to know when it would happen, so I packed up my hammock and started getting all of my stored bags off the support boat so I'd be ready to leave at short notice. Once that was done it was just a matter of waiting.

RACE DAY – STAGE 5

As the morning wore on, my mind played an emotional see-saw with the pro's and con's of dropping out of the last two stages of the race. While my overriding feeling was one of disappointment at quitting, I couldn't help but be relieved at not having to go on.

One of my concerns about doing the long stage was that I would lose track of the route marker tape and get lost, and given that the reliability of the markings was of a concern in the shorter stages, made me think that, over 108km, it is sure to be a huge problem. *And…*we would be trying to spot it in the *dark!* With last minute changes to the course having to be done now, there was an even greater chance there would be lengthy gaps between markers, which would spell disaster for someone with as bad a sense of direction as what I have.

Also, another two days and nights of eating dehydrated food and sleeping in a hammock lined with sand, were yet more arguments to convince myself I was doing the right thing.

Yet the word "quitter" still rang loud in my ears as I looked over to see Kim laying in her hammock with her bandaged feet resting over the edge. She wouldn't have finished Stage 4 until well into the evening last night, after being on the track for over 13 ½ hours, yet here she was, determined to continue on and line up at the start line for Stage 5. As I started talking to her, she told me she also suffered from chaffing around the top of her legs and she had slid her hand down there and applied some "BodyGlide" to it, in an attempt to lubricate the friction hotspot. Her ultra-endurance experience had certainly prepared her better for this type of event than what my experience had.

I asked if she was still planning to do all six stages and she replied: "Well that's what I came here for so I may as well do it". Now I *really* felt like a quitter! Here I was, not a single blister on my feet and just a little bit of crotch rash, and I had given up. In fact, I'd given up before I'd even developed the crotch rash! I was in awe of this lady's strength and determination. Jacquie Palmer (US), Kim's companion for much of the race, was also still in the race, and prepared to do whatever it would take to finish what she started.

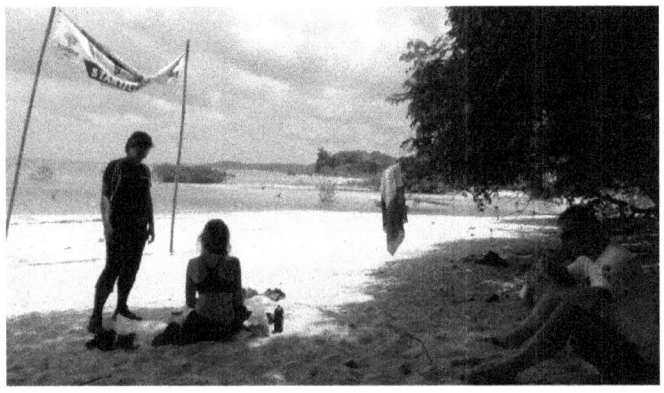

I stayed close to the other people who were planning to go to Santarem so I didn't miss any news of a departure time. In the meantime, I changed into a clean set of clothes that were in my main luggage bags, and despite still not having had a shower, I felt considerably better once I took the smelly camp clothes off. A morning dunk in the river helped wash some of the jungle filth off me but nothing was going to feel as good as the first shower I would have when I finally got to a hotel.

RACE DAY – STAGE 5

The clean shorts I put on had gone from comfortably close-fitting to loose fitting in the 6 days I had been in the jungle. I estimated I had probably lost about 3kg in weight over that time, and I shuddered at the thought of how much more weight I would lose if I was to do the 108km stage. I felt good though. Apart from the muscle aches in my upper back, I had survived the four days of racing without anything more serious than a bit of chaffing on my upper legs and lower back. I doubted there were many other people – if any – who got this far without a single blister on their feet or black toenail.

The word finally came that our lift to Santarem had arrived so we carried our bags up to the track where the two vehicles were waiting for us. There were ten people checking out and we all had to squeeze into just two old dual-cab utilities.

The back trays of both vehicles were overloaded with bags, and with no cover to hold them in while driving over the rough dirt road, I was worried some of the bags may not make it to Santarem. I was glad my bags were in the first car so if they fell out, there was a chance the second car would see them on the road.

We split into two groups of five, with one person sitting in the front with the driver, and the remaining four people squeezing into the back seats of each car. Being the smallest in our car I volunteered to sit on the other peoples knees as we crumpled up in the small space.

The drive to Santarem took about an hour, half of that on a pot-holed dirt road and the rest on a sealed road. My sense of guilt at deserting the rest of the group was eased somewhat by the fact that so many others were doing the same, and I also felt we were probably doing Shirley a favor by leaving her with less people to try and manage under the difficult circumstances.

When we got to the outskirts of Santarem there was a sense of relief that we were finally back in civilization. But we weren't quite there yet. To our surprise the Brazilian driver pulled up in front of a train station and gestured for us to get out.

As I had come to expect, the Brazilian driver didn't understand any English and we made futile efforts to ask him to take us to the hotel we were booked into for the finish of the race. Finally I was able to get him to understand when I said the name of the hotel. We were so relieved when we recognized his "ah-ha" moment and he smiled approvingly at us as he ushered us back into his car. It was only a few more minutes before we were driving up the winding ramp into the reception area of the Barrudada Tropical Hotel, where we would stay until we met up with the rest of the runners after they completed the remaining two stages of the race.

Finally Stage 5 Begins

With the amended start time now 2pm, the race organizers prepared the alternative course with marker tape and set up checkpoints with crews of medics and race volunteers. With the level of support from her local Brazilian crew noticeably compromised after the disqualification of the local runner, Shirley was relying heavily on the medical team for reliable assistance.

RACE DAY – STAGE 5

The local core team that Shirley paid to help with the organizing of the event didn't seem to acknowledge the potential danger of using the existing route. Despite being given instructions to remark parts of the course and put boats and equipment in place, and then confirming it was all done, it eventually became apparent that a lot of this wasn't done.

After wasting a lot of valuable daylight hours, Stage 5 finally started at 2pm. Even the fastest runners now faced running through most of the night and it would take until nearly 4pm the next day before the last of the competitors would finally cross the finish line.

To avoid having to run through the section of jungle where the disqualified runner lived, the runners were to be transported by a small boat around this area. The boat would shuttle groups of people around the compromised zone and the runners would then continue on the marked route through the jungle.

The communication between Shirley and the key people on the support staff was practically non-existent, with them not responding to her on the radio, supposedly because they were in an area that didn't have radio coverage. It was almost impossible for the race director to know what was going on along the long 108km of the Stage 5 course and the medics proved to be the only reliable source of information.

Time was not on the runners side now and they couldn't afford to stop and sleep because they would not have made it to the finish line before it got dark for the second night.

Having not covered the Stage 5 course myself, I was interested to hear the experiences from the runners who did do it.

Jacquie Palmer, from New York, struggled with the difficult conditions and poorly marked course for over 25 hours, with just a catnap of a rest in all that time. Her story is a remarkable testament to her determination to not give in to the extreme physical and mental fatigue she would have been experiencing while in the jungle. Here is her amazing account of "the long stage":

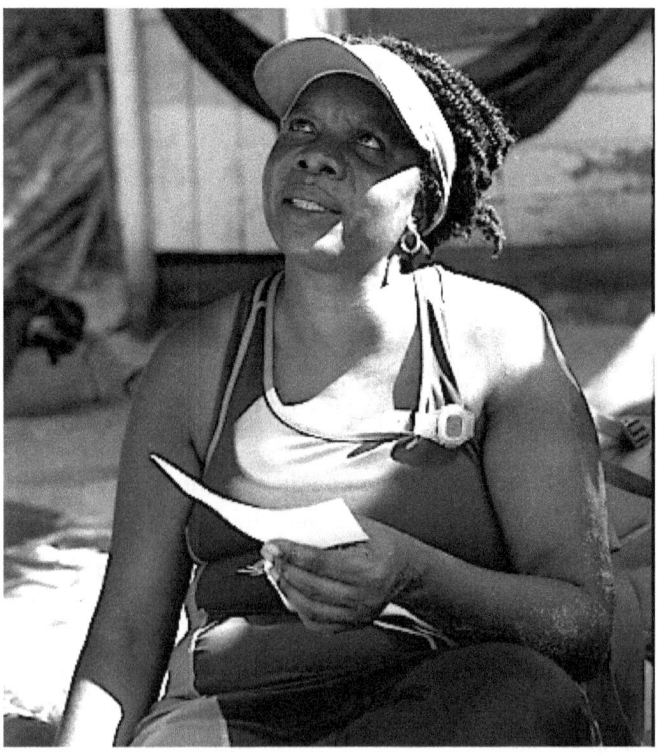

RACE DAY – STAGE 5

"I will always remember the long stage of the race distinctly. The stage started late due to issues the day before and instead of the scheduled 5 am start we started at 2pm in the blazing sun. The first 3 miles or so was on rough, hilly and unshaded clay road with sharp rocks although sometimes the soil would change to pure sand. The fluctuation in the surface on one stretch of road was a bit crazy. I could see dark clouds in the sky and my nose was itching for the smell of rain. As a child of the West Indies it's second nature to smell rain even before it begins to pour. The rain did come but in halting big drops, providing little relief from the sun.

I was keeping up with Kim which was a good sign. As we made our way into the jungle, the trail was freshly created with short steep up climbs. More roots to hang on to than the first stage but just as hilly and breathless as Stage 1. The jungle was not as dark as the other stages but we made a few wrong turns due to missing tags. I met two runners who said they were going in circles due to missing tags also.

The long stage shifted from jungle to long lonely rocky road with hardly any contact with other humans except for the now and then single motorcyclist. When night fell I was transported by a small boat (about a 20 minute ride) to another long lonely stretch of road. I don't even know what time it was but I was falling asleep as I was walking. I could feel myself veering off to the side of the road as my eyes closed involuntarily. I remember forcing myself to sing the Chaka Khan song "I'm every woman" over and over and over again just to stay awake.

I hated the doctors on the long section; they would not allow me to rest. They rushed me through the check points insisting that I need to catch the ride on the boat and the other runners were waiting for me. Bullshit…..that boat must have left me already! I was tired, I was seeing mirages. 11 hours into the long stage I came to one of the bigger check points. Shirley's boat was docked fully lighted and I longed to climb aboard and sleep. My feet were burning, blisters were all over them and the bandage was of no use. At this point I just wanted to sleep. This was the first time since starting the long section that I would be eating. I devoured the full bag of stew beans without even a thought that I just had two servings instead of one.

Shirley came over and told me that I had a deep river crossing in the dark. I started to cry....I couldn't do a river crossing at this time of the night. She must have felt sorry for me because she told me to go aboard the boat and let John wrap my feet and to take a nap. I fell asleep while John worked on protecting my feet. Maybe about an hour later John woke me up and told me that Shirley had arranged a boat ride for me. This was such a relief. This was my second boat ride for the night. It was a short ride and then I had to take another boat ride which took about an hour across the river. Even though it was a low speed boat and I was being soaked wet I felt as if I was being transported to a different world. From the boat level everything was dark on the river but when you turned towards the sky the stars felt as if they were right at my fingertips. Shooting stars were just blasting across the sky in the numbers. I started to make "wishes". After the boat ride I walked another long lonely road which eventually turning into a sandy section that was leading to the river. Glow sticks were on the trail floor making it easy to navigate.

Eventually, I came to the river in the dark. Bull frogs were all over the beach. Every step I took a frog came leaping towards or away from me. Oh my god....freakily scary. From then on to the end of the long section it was beach.

The first stretch of beach of about 3 miles or so was bordered with large black rock formations that had a hidden exit. I say hidden because around 5am that morning I saw Kim and Antonio making their way towards me on the beach. They explained that they had walked to the tip of the rocks and couldn't figure out how to go around it. I knew I was going in the right direction so I said let's try together. The exit looks hidden from a distance but when you climb across the rocks it was open to the other side of the beach. This was a difficult climb because the rocks were all over the beach and especially with aching and hurt feet it felt like hell going through this section.

We had several river crossings in order to get to the other side. It was either walking through the river or climbing ridiculously enormous rocks and in some cases we didn't have a choice except to walk into the river to the other side of the beach."

- Jacquie Palmer

******

Kim Frankish (UK) was another of the four women in the remaining stages of the 254km event who battled with sleep deprivation, sore feet and missing marker tape to eventually complete the long stage. Here is her story:

"The late start actually helped me because it gave me more time to recover from the long previous day when I didn't reach the camp until around 11pm.

I set off with Antonio (from Italy), who I had walked with on an earlier stage. The early part of the stage passed fairly unremarkably. When we finally got to the first of the river crossings we had to run for the boat to cross the river and I literally flew down the bank. My legs couldn't keep up with my head and I fell head first in the sand. Luckily it was dark and no one saw me but the important thing was we caught the boat!

The trip across was cold and uncomfortable as most of the space had already been taken. Arriving at the other side it was straight off the boat and more or less straight into a water crossing. The bulk of runners were soon out of sight but Antonio and I kept going at a comfortable pace.

Some of the ribbons were hard to find in the dark and several times we had to retrace our steps. Due to my late arrival in camp the night before, I had missed the briefing and wasn't aware that there weren't going to be any markers and we were to keep to the beach. Fortunately we eventually came across a small boat that was to take us back across the river. It was a fantastic trip, it was cold but the sky was black and full of stars, I have never seen so many!

We set off again and had another water crossing sometime later but because it was so dark we had to be taken across in a boat to avoid the chance of running into anacondas or caiman.

Most of the night we just seemed to be trudging along tracks which seem to go on for ever. Finally we reached a check point on the beach. There was a small fire so we stopped for forty winks. It was really cold and I had stupidly given Shirley my merino top and bottoms which I now regretted as a big mistake. It started to get light so we set off and walked the full length of the beach but I was worried we hadn't seen any markers so persuaded Antonio to retrace our steps.

We were happy to eventually met up with Jacqui and the bombeiros and be told we were heading in the right direction. My feet were very cold and hurt sooo much by now I could hardly walk and I just lost all my enthusiasm and felt really dejected. I had lost all coordination and was running on empty.

Antonio headed off and once I was on my own I really struggled. I couldn't get my act together and even tried to sing some of my favourite songs but couldn't remember any words!

With sheer determination I finally completed the long stage. I couldn't wait for my last night in a hammock as I really enjoyed

RACE DAY – STAGE 5

sleeping in it, especially the nights we could hear the howler monkeys. We all hung up our light sticks in the camp - what a lovely sight.

Waking up the next morning, for the start of Stage 6, I was amazed at what a difference a day makes. I intended to enjoy every km and every minute of this final stage. There were rocky bits and mangroves which were tough but the sun and the locals made it a wonderful stage. A little boy ran over with 2 bottles of water which brought tears to my eyes. The part I enjoyed most was the final river crossing – I loved it (I don't do water as I don't swim). Then we were back on the beach, around some rocks and there was the finish line - it had come sooner than I expected. What a fantastic journey - and the ice cream mmmm just topped it off.

Why is it that when you finish your feet really let you know what you have put them through. Although I didn't suffer from any blisters my feet were very macerated from being wet so much but a few days of pain brings a life time of memories- plus you meet some fantastic people!"

- Kim Frankish

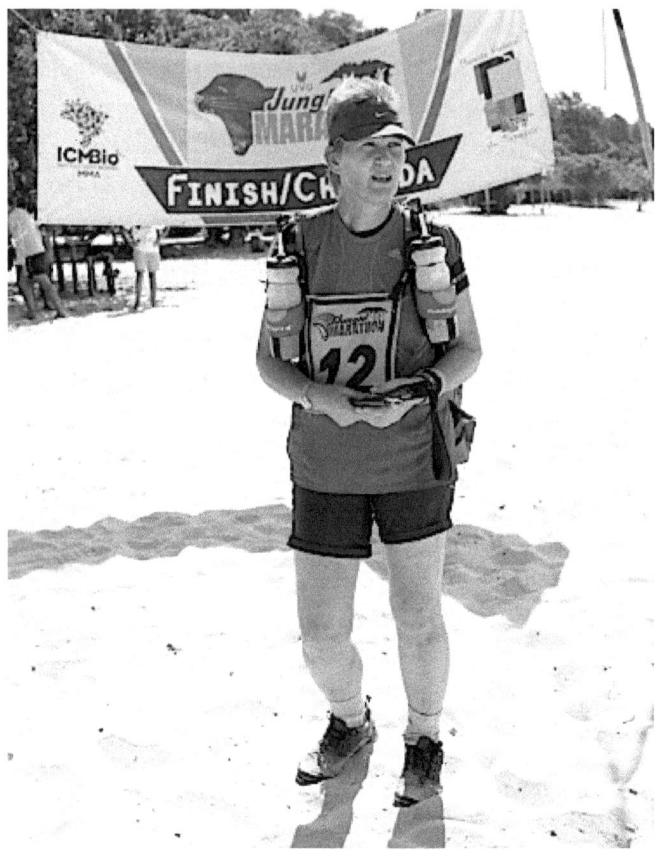

Jacquie, Kim and Antonio would cross the finish line of Stage 5 after a staggering non-stop 25 hours and 20 minutes in the jungle - but they wouldn't be the only ones to experience problems navigating the amended course.

A group of four runners got lost – *really lost* – and ended up in Santarem! None of them spoke Portuguese, but ingeniously they managed to get the telephone number of ICMBio off the logo on the front of their race pamphlet and phoned them to find out where the finish line was. They arrived at the finish line from the opposite direction to where they were supposed to come from and covered many more miles than the rest of the long stage runners. Their frustratingly long journey took them 21 hours and 27 minutes and had them tramping through the jungle all night with just the light from their headlamps illuminating the tracks and not knowing which direction they should have been travelling in once they lost sight of the marker tape.

There was no doubt the last minute changes to the Stage 5 route compromised the runner's ability to negotiate it. With the start time being over 9 hours later in the day than originally planned, it meant the runners had to run in darkness through areas that were previously expected to be covered in the light of day. For eight years the "*dark zone*" had been a pre-determined area that could be strategically compensated for to allow the competitors to safely navigate it during the night, but the new dark zone had now become as unpredictable as the violent race threats themselves.

Rushed changes to the plans by exhausted organizers, led to botched changes to the course in some places, which then resulted in many people getting lost. Even having clear markings cannot guarantee people will easily follow them. The combination of fatigue and darkness would make following the marked route very difficult.

******

Alfredo DiMeo, an Italian who now lives in the UK,

was one of the runners who also had problems in Stage 5. His story is just as incredible as Jacquie's and gives an insight into the arduous task the competitors faced to get to the finish line. Here is Alfredo's account of the long stage:

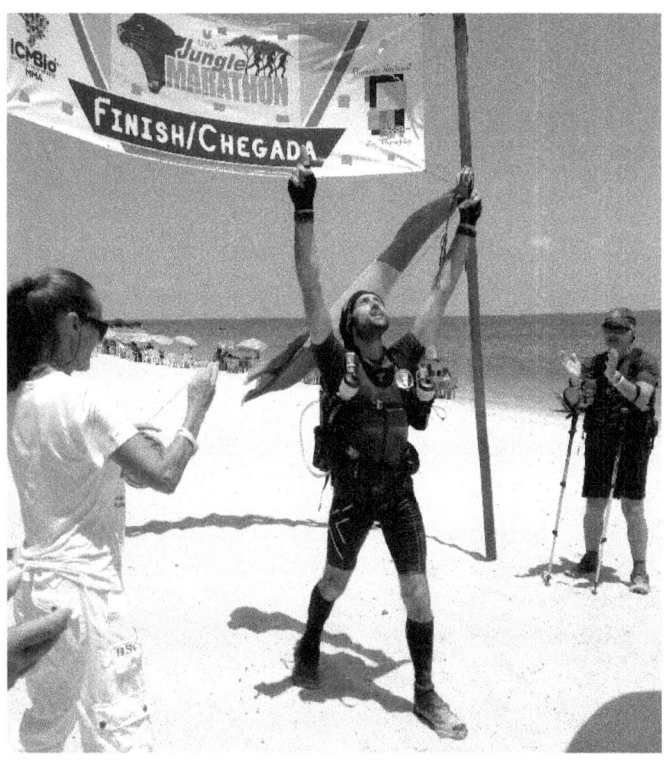

"After the confusion surrounding the disqualification of the athlete caught cheating, the delayed start to the long stage of the race proved to be less beneficial to myself. The extra 12 hours of resting allowed my body and mental presence to relax a little too much!

I felt sluggish and lethargic at the start and not really up for the stage. This loss of mental approach and interest for the race proved to

RACE DAY – STAGE 5

be a turning point in my race that was costly.

5km into the stage my loss of concentration on the trail caused myself, and an American competitor behind me, to miss the course marker entirely which resulted in us both exiting an area of deep jungle onto a road that we had previously run down......or was it up ?

There were red course markers to the left and to the right of us. Which direction should we take? Immediate option was to run towards the marker down hill and see if we could see somebody around the corner. Everything looked familiar and what we had not realized was that we had run this section approximately 20 minutes before. It was then that we saw the foot prints running in the opposite direction to what we were heading downhill from, which posed another set of questions - were these from the people in front of us? Or were these ours from previously?

Confusion, anger and frustration set in over the next 30 minutes as we admitted there was a problem and that we were lost, with nobody around to help. This lack of contact with race officials was the trigger for the anger.

Matt, the American guy, suggested that we retrace our steps, which would be easy enough if we knew where we had exited – but every hole in the jungle cover looked the same. Matt would dive back into the jungle but only as far at any one period that I could still see him and keep in vocal contact with him.

Eventually after over an hour a vehicle carrying race staff passed and we hailed them down, alas they were useless as none spoke English or seemed in any way interested in helping. We decided to follow the direction they were traveling in and for 20 minutes we did so, following sporadic training shoe prints in the sandy dust. It was then that we recognized a break in the jungle that we had entered over 2 hours ago.

We were extremely frustrated and low on water as we tried to make up lost ground. We eventually caught up with the last placed competitor with her Brazilian guide so we knew we were heading towards the next checkpoint. I had lost interest in the race, and confidence in the race organization. I had mentally decided to quit at the next checkpoint which was ironically at the base camp that I had left earlier that morning.

Matt had gone off ahead on my instruction, as I had told him of my decision to quit. I arrived at the checkpoint and vented my anger at the lack of information and support out on the trail. It was wrong to do so as they were volunteers, not race officials, and they had also been trying to battle with the last minute changes to the course. Matt was there and he urged me to continue and not give up as it was only 12 miles to the boat that we had to rendezvous with.

His appeal worked as 12 miles was the distance from Victoria Park in East London to Tower Bridge which I had run many times over the last 3 years and I knew it was nothing as the crow flew.

We left together both refreshed and positive........it took us into the jungle during late afternoon and into the darkness. It was my first experience of running in a jungle environment in the dark, and the rules completely change with paranoia and fatigue playing their part.

Reaching a swamp and river crossing 5 miles from the rendezvous point of the boat in the darkness was an unforgettable experience, putting ones fears and doubts into perspective, forcing you to follow your trust and instincts amassed in all the years of your running career.

I will never forget arriving in the dark to this crossing and having to enter the water and feeling the weeds and vegetation around my body as I began to swim towards the other side. Looking back now, it was crazy, as I will never know what was in there.

Making the boat was a chance to refuel and rest and then mentally prepare for the grueling remainder of the stage that would take us into the next day.

I guess the point to appreciate about the experience was that simple mistakes can be made when you are tired and under pressure. Sometimes we choose to see things and make choices that are not always the correct ones. However there is always a solution as long as you keep the desire and will to succeed in your heart.

I sum up that the fear of failure during the race spurred me on. We are all afraid of failure."

- Alfredo DiMeo

******

UK competitor **Anthony Hugill** managed to avoid any major dramas on the Stage 5 course, with his military and ultra-endurance experience helping him to avoid losing any time from getting lost. His account of the long stage highlights how important it was to have the company of other runners when the going got tough.

Despite the fact that long distance running is a highly individual sport, there was no doubt that everyone who participated in the Jungle Marathon found added strength when in the company of other runners who would help pace and encourage each other to keep going. Here is Anthony's account of the long stage:

"I set off at a decent pace after the delayed start and made it to the boat pick up area in 12th or 13th place. The boat took me to the drop-off point and I went for it, running behind two guys one of which one was Argentinian. They were both good runners and we covered some ground, pulling away from the main group we were on the boat

with.

We arrived at the river crossing but had to wait to be picked up by some small raider type boats. We waited for about half an hour until the main group who were with us on the boat started to filter in to the assembly area. We crossed the river in one boat with another boat breaking down.

When we reached the other side of the river I set off by myself this time and was by myself while running through the night, which I liked in a strange way - just me and the jungle and the odd tracks.

I reached another checkpoint after a short river crossing and warmed myself up by a fire. After refilling my water bottles I set off again, leaving the checkpoint with a few others. We headed down a beach but after a good while of no light sticks or markers I started to doubt myself and wondered if I had taken a wrong turn.

I looked back and could see more runners so I thought this must be right and my instinct told me to just keep going. I kept to the waterline and after about 4 or 5 miles I found a light stick floating in the water so knew I must have been on the right track. I also kept picking up foot prints of running shoes so felt confident I was heading in the right direction.

Shortly after first light broke I reached another checkpoint. After running along the beach again for some time I made out three figures of a woman and two men behind me and was relieved to finally see someone else. The two men were Brazilian competitors Regis Botter and Ricardo da Silva and we joined up and went for it.

Regis was a hard man - his feet had swelled so badly he cut the toes off each trainer and ran with his toes poking out, through thorns and jungle undergrowth, and never once flinched.

We helped each other through a swampy lagoon which seemed never ending. Regis and Ricardo really helped me get through the later part of the stage and I found them both to be incredibly good people.

RACE DAY – STAGE 5

After hitting the beach again we could just make out the finish line which was still a good 3 or 4 miles off but we were relieved to finally be finishing.

I must say that the Jungle Marathon has to be one of the hardest events I have ever done in respect of the climate and terrain. I have completed a 160 mile desert ultra single stage but the jungle was something else, and the people and competitors second to none. I did it to help raise funds for charity and it was well worth it."

- Anthony Hugill

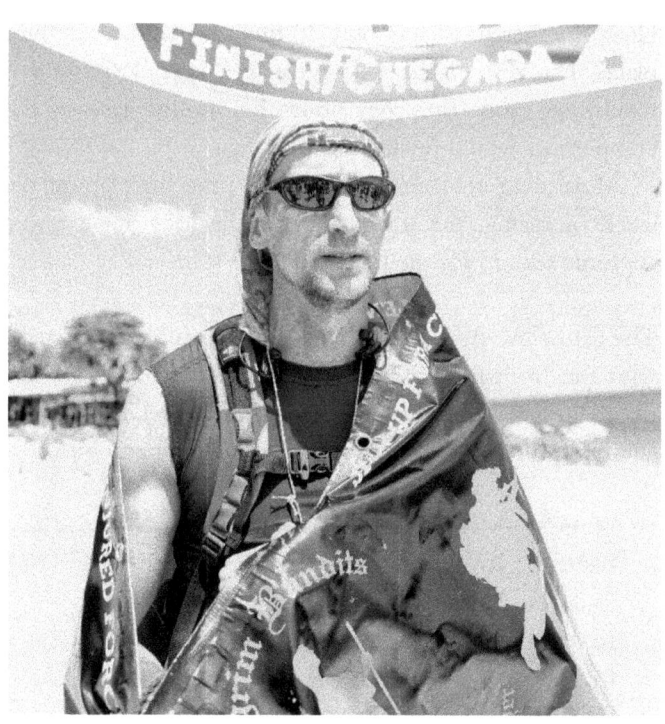

Stage 5 Race Summary

Everyone who lined up at the start of Stage 5 eventually completed the dreaded "long stage". The last minute changes to the route kept both the organizers and the competitors on their toes and left the race director battling to coordinate the widely dispersed parties over the 108km of extreme terrain.

Marcelo Sinoca (Brazil) was the first to cross the finish line in a remarkable time of 14:35:14 and was followed by Rodrigo Souza (Brazil) only a few minutes later. Sebastian Haag (Netherlands) was only 20 minutes behind for third place. The rest of the field were well spread out and it would be more than ten hours before the last of the competitors would finally finish.

More than any other moment in time throughout the week of racing, the finish line for the long stage is the supreme reward for the few who make it there.

The list below shows the time taken to complete the stage, with the front-runners pushing themselves to their limits of endurance, and the competitors trailing behind them surviving set-backs that ultimately tested their resolve.

    14:35:14   Marcelo Sinoca (Brazil)
    14:39:14   Rodrigo Souza (Brazil)
    15:00:14   Sebastian Haag (Germany)
    16:00:51   Gustavo Rodrigues (Brazil)
    16:23:50   Alex Vicintin (Brazil)
    16:23:52   Roberto Ameiro (Brazil)
    18:13:47   Mario Angel Oyola (Argentina)
    18:15:05   Jerlison Almeida (Brazil)

RACE DAY – STAGE 5

18:15:06 Eder Morimoto (Brazil)
18:59:30 Jason Wolfe (USA)
19:03:35 Regis Botter (Brazil)
          Anthony Hugill (UK)
          Ricardo da Silva (Brazil)
19:07:56 Jacqueline Terto (Brazil)
19:12:20 Jean-Paul Van Der Bas (Netherlands)
19:12:38 Geovane Rento de Carvalho (Brazil)
19:18:20 Krzysztof Sobczak (Poland)
19:30:20 Lien Choong Luen (Singapore)
21:26:57 Marcelo Vanzuita (NZ)
          Alfredo DiMeo (UK)
          Cleber Evangelista (Brazil)
21:54:30 Jereon Roodenburg (Netherlands)
21:59:12 Petter Vallestad (Norway)
          Berndt Tvedt (Norway)
22:50:21 Moon-Ka Leung (China)
          Matt Buck (USA)
          Marie Ann Danet (France)
22:51:11 Pedro Vera Jimenez (Venezuela)
25:18:08 Antonio Gianella (Italy)
25:20:50 Kim Frankish (UK)
25:20:55 Jacquie Palmer (USA)

(Females are in italics)

Chapter 10

RACE DAY – STAGE 6

Pajucara to Maracana Beach, Santarem – 14.5km

Stage 6 Brief

There will be no checkpoints on this final shorter stage.

After spending two nights in a comfortable bed and a day sight-seeing with some of the other runners who had finished the Jungle Marathon after Stage 4, I was happy to be back in civilization, well fed and well rested.

The designated Jungle Marathon hotel in Santarem, the Barrudada Tropical Hotel, was quite an impressive establishment considering the standard of the city buildings it was surrounded by.

Santarem is the second most important city in the state of Para, in Northern Brazil, and lies on the banks of the Tapajos where it joins the Amazon River. Founded in 1661, the city now has a population of approximately 300,000.

The city blocks surrounding the hotel were a mixture of very old housing and relatively modern shopping centres with the pot-holed streets having what appeared to

RACE DAY – STAGE 6

be open sewage drains running along them. The dense tropical air absorbed the unsanitary urban odours and left me appreciating the lush tropical rainforest that I had been cursing only days before.

Despite the relatively poor neighborhood, the hotel was quite luxurious with a beautiful outdoor dining area that faced out onto an invitingly refreshing swimming pool.

Like all the other places I had been to on my way through Brazil no-one here spoke any English, or very little, so it was difficult communicating with the restaurant and bar staff. After eventually figuring out how to ask for steak, chips and beer I gladly stuck with those three menu items for the duration of my stay. After spending seven days in the jungle eating only dehydrated food, steak, chips and beer had never tasted so good!

The second morning of our stay at the Barrudada Tropical Hotel would see the final stage of the Jungle Marathon finishing at a nearby beach along the Tapajos River. Maracana Beach in Santarem was the location of the finish line for Stage 6 for the competitors who were still yet to finish the 254km Jungle Marathon event.

Those of us who were already in Santarem were unsure about what time the runners were expected to start arriving at the finish line and as the final stage was only a short one, we decided to be at the beach by 9am so we wouldn't miss the first of the athletes to cross the line.

The taxi ride was long and tortuous over the most potholed roads I had ever driven along. The road leading down to the beach seemed to go on forever and was in such a bad state of disrepair the taxi could only travel at a snails pace as it swerved around crater-sized holes in the neglected old bitumen roads.

The urban area consisted predominantly of dilapidated shanty homes that border-lined on third-world standards but as we got closer to the beach there were many blocks that appeared to have modern tourist accommodation being built on them, which was in stark contrast to the surrounding dwellings.

The road seemed to go from bad to worse and I started to worry that the driver was taking us into some sort of ghetto rather than to the idyllic-sounding Maracana Beach. It was only after the road seemed to come to an end in front of us, and shanty café's replaced the shanty houses, that I started to relax.

After finally reaching the river we drove along a rough track that took us past the back entrances of the café's that lined Maracana Beach. We paid the taxi driver and walked down to the beach to see if we could find anyone else involved with the Jungle Marathon.

The café staff were only just starting to set up their chairs in the sand out the front of the buildings as we arrived. There was no sign of the finish line banner but we could see a group of people a little further up the beach so we walked up to join them. It wasn't long before the crowd of people grew as the family and friends of the local Brazilian competitors gathered to watch the final hours of the 2013 Jungle Marathon.

The TV Globo film crew arrived and started setting up their equipment so they could be ready to capture the final moments of the race on film. The drone camera sprung to life above us, captivating everyone on the beach who

RACE DAY – STAGE 6

hadn't seen it before.

It wasn't long before the race organizers had arrived and erected the finish line banner on two lengths of timber dug into the sand. The growing crowd of spectators who had congregated at the nearby beachside bar was growing more excited in anticipation of seeing the first of the Jungle Marathon runners cross the finish line.

******

After completing the long stage the day before, all the runners had a chance to rest overnight before starting the 6th and final stage of the 245km event. Having the long stage as the second to last stage enables everyone to finish the last stage of the race spaced out over just a couple of hours instead of over 10 hours.

Although Stage 6 was originally meant to be over 20km, it had been shortened to about 14.5km after the camp location at the end of Stage 5 ended up being closer to Santarem than it should have been due to the last-minute changes to the course.

With this stage being much shorter than the rest, and no checkpoints having to be provided, many of the volunteers, medics and runners who had already dropped out from the previous stages, ran the course in a gesture of solidarity for the weary competitors who were about to finally complete their Jungle Marathon challenge.

For the runners themselves, this final stage was a mere formality as the previous stages had produced a gap of over two hours between the first and second runner and this gap couldn't be closed over the short distance of the final stage. With this in mind the first three place getters, along with a few other runners, would run the stage as a group and plan to cross the finish line together. The competitive spirit didn't serve any purpose now and instead, it was time to unite and celebrate the coming to a close of an amazing race and enjoy the camaraderie of the fellow competitors, many of whom would probably be life-long friends from this moment on.

Today was the day to put all the race politics aside and revel in the anticipation of completing the worlds toughest endurance race.

******

The large group of family, friends and fellow runners waiting at the finish line at Maracana Beach cheered as the first of the runners could be seen running down from the rocky outcrops at the far end of the beach.

As one competitor started the final stretch along the sandy bank of the Tapajos River towards the finish line another could be seen following close behind him up on the rocks. The race photographers, film crew and spectators crowded onto the beach behind the finish line with their cameras on the ready to capture the moment of victorious relief as each runner completed their final stage of the grueling ultra-endurance race.

Shirley was also there to present them with their well-earned medal. After placing it around their neck, she handed them a refreshing ice-cream to help cool them down.

Although the medals for the 127km event and 254km event looked the same, the latter one was much bigger and reflected the much greater achievement these runners had completed.

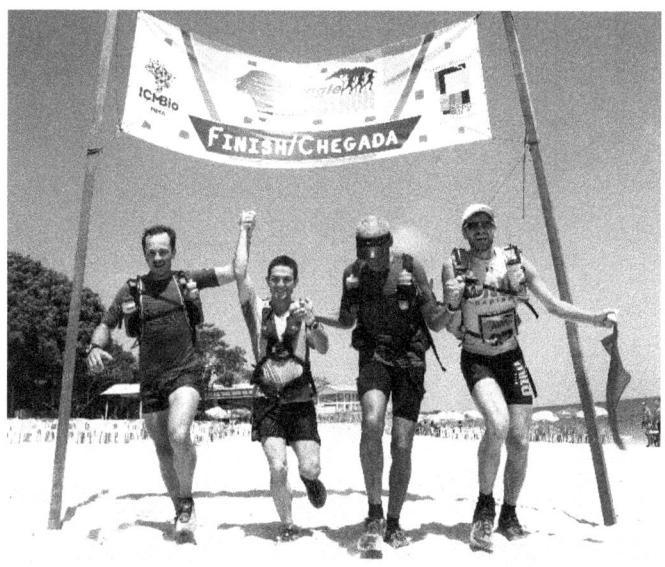

Three runners crossed the finish line with only a minute separating them all and they were then followed by a group of seven running close together, three of whom would be the eventual overall first, second and third place getters for this years Jungle Marathon.

Marcelo Sinoca (Brazil) had claimed first place victory in a total race time of 32:18:14 for the six stages. His time placed him over an hour ahead of the second place getter, Rodrigo Souza (Brazil), and two hours ahead of Sebastian Haag (Germany) who finished third overall.

Half an hour later the first of the female runners crossed the finish line and was overcome with emotion as Shirley placed the large, locally made ceramic Jungle Marathon medal around her neck. Jacquie Terto (Brazil) had claimed her third victory in the 245km Jungle Marathon and couldn't have been happier!

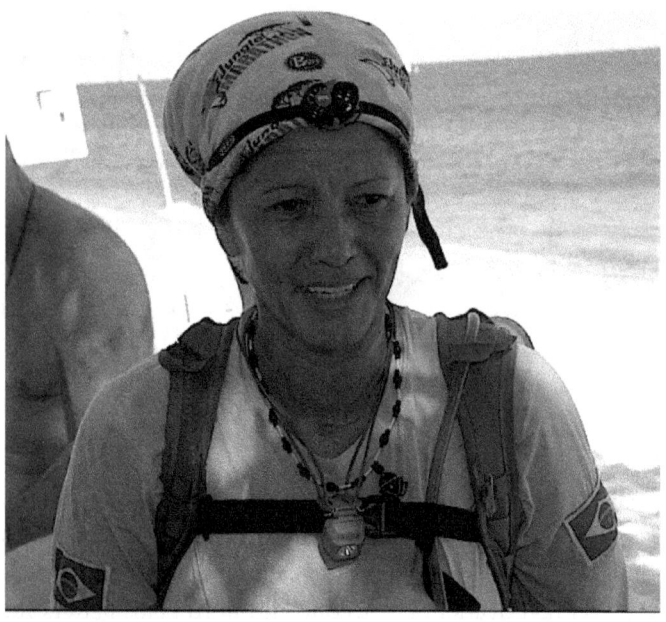

Jacquie's total time of 45:55:33 for the 6 stages placed her as the first woman in the 254km event and 14th position overall. She had now won the 254km event three times and the 127km event once - an amazing achievement! She could now relax and bask in the glory of being the Jungle Marathon Queen.

RACE DAY – STAGE 6

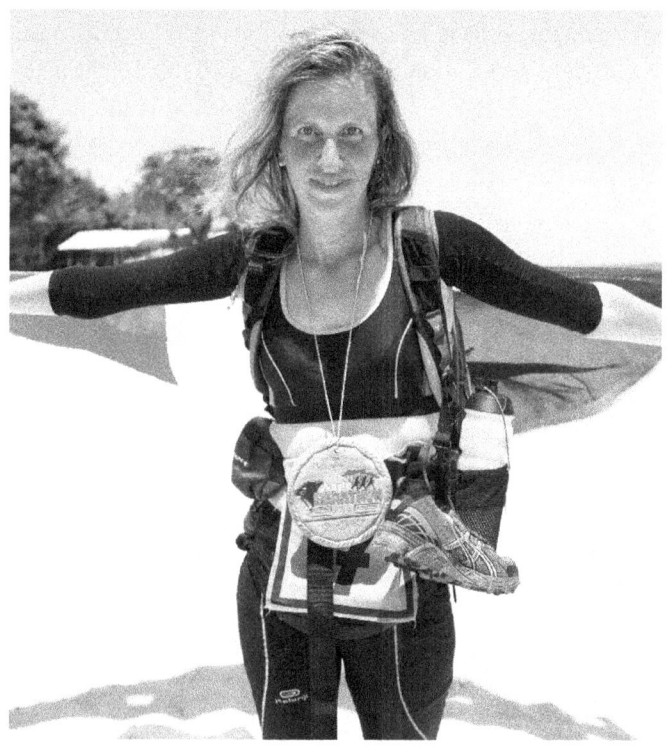

Marie Ann Danet (France) claimed second place out of the women followed by Kim Frankish (UK) and Jacquie Palmer (USA). They were all now proud owners of 254km Jungle Marathon finishers medal!

Once all the competitors had crossed the finish line it was time to celebrate. Lunch was provided for all the Jungle Marathon competitors, volunteers and staff at the beachside bar that we had all been sitting in while waiting for the runners to arrive at Maracana Beach. There was no denying there were some very hungry people in this crowd. This would be the first time in 9 days that the 254km event runners would have fresh food and ice cold beverages and the delight showed on their faces as they piled their plates high with food from the smorgasbord spread of local cuisine.

After everyone had finished eating it was time to collect all the luggage that had been stored on the riverboat for the duration of the race and climb aboard one of the two chartered coaches that would take us all back to the Tropical Barrudada Hotel in Santarem.

The ride back into town was even more uncomfortable in the bus than what it had been in the taxi. With many of the pot-holes being too large for the buses to drive around they had to instead slow down to a crawling pace and drive through them. There was no breaking the jovial spirit of the runners though and just knowing they were on their way to a clean hotel room with hot and cold running water was worth putting up with the bumpy ride.

Frozen ice blocks were passed around to everyone on the bus and we all sucked on the home-made plastic tubes of frozen juice as the over-crowded bus jostled it's way towards the hotel. There was no denying that most of the people on the bus definitely needed a shower. Nine days of jungle stench was going to take some scrubbing to get off these race-weary bodies.

After arriving at the hotel we had a few hours for the runners to get settled into their rooms and freshen up. At 5:30pm we would be climbing aboard another bus that would take us to the riverside restaurant where we would enjoy our celebration dinner and the medal presentations for the overall first, second and third place getters in each of the events.

Many of the people made their way to the inviting swimming pool for a swim or enjoyed a cold beer in the adjoining outside dining area. It was now time to relax and start the process of adjusting back into civilization.

Chapter 11

THE PRESENTATION DINNER

At 5:30pm two chartered buses departed the Barrudada Tropical Hotel for the restaurant where the Jungle Marathon dinner and presentation ceremony would be held. It was strange to see everybody in clean casual clothes and smelling like soap instead of swamp. The atmosphere was jovial and relaxed and you could sense the feeling of relief at finally having the race completed. The hard work was done and all that was left now was to celebrate.

The drive out to the restaurant seemed to take forever. After driving for about 20 minutes along bitumen roads the bus took a left turn onto a sandy track that narrowed down to a single lane. The road was mostly loose sand and in many places I was surprised that the bus didn't get bogged down in the loose surface. It gently rolled from side to side as it negotiated the changing contours of the jungle track and relied heavily on the harder surface along the wheel ruts from previous traffic to keep it from sinking into the sand. There were very few places for vehicles coming from the opposite direction to pass and on a couple of occasions vehicles coming towards us had to reverse back to a wider section of the road so both vehicles could continue on their way.

After driving for about half an hour along the sandy track we finally arrived at the restaurant. The buses pulled into the car park and everyone shuffled off and headed into the charming tropical setting of the popular restaurant.

The Jungle Marathon presentation dinner is held at the Casa de Saulo Restaurant every year. Set high up on a cliff overlooking the Tapajos River it is the perfect location to complete our jungle experience. With the sun about to set below the horizon I took the opportunity to walk down the timber staircase in front of the restaurant gardens to explore the expansive fluvial beach along the river before the fading twilight left it all in darkness. I joined a number of other tourists who had already positioned themselves to capture the majestic sight of the sun setting below the horizon over the mighty river. This was my last chance to enjoy the amazing Amazon tributary and the sunset made for the perfect final photo.

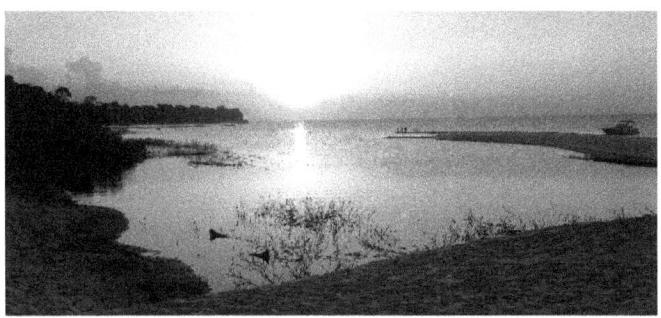

Once back up at the restaurant, I noticed there were complimentary glasses of a popular local cocktail laid out on a trestle table in between the building that housed the bar and kitchen and the large open-aired dining area. In between the buildings and the cliff face there was a lovely garden with a well maintained lawn and a small swimming pool surrounded by timber decking and outdoor settings that were now occupied by the relaxing guests. This was a jungle experience I could get use to!

As the time wore on everyone was getting very hungry and anxious to start eating and although everyone had been at the restaurant for some time there was no sign of Shirley, the race director. Despite this, the buffet dishes were spread out on a table in the dining area and everyone lined up to get their meal.

The sight of all the food laid out in front of us stirred up more lively chatter as everyone patiently waited for their turn to pile their plate high with the many dishes on offer. For most of the people it would be their first decent feed in over nine grueling days.

Once everyone had finished their meal it was time to start the presentations - but where was Shirley? She still hadn't been seen and no-one seemed to know where she was. With the medal presentations about to commence an announcement was made that Shirley couldn't make it and Basti Haag, who was not only one of the competitors but also a representative for the sponsoring company UVU, would be presenting the awards on her behalf.

Everyone thought it extraordinary that Shirley didn't join us not only for dinner but also for the all-important awards ceremony. While Basti did a great job it just didn't feel right. But everyone still had a great evening and enjoyed our last hours as a united group before the first of the marathoners would start the exodus out of Santarem Airport and back to their home countries in the early hours of the morning. The next 24 hours would see all of the competitors, medics and international volunteer crew fly back to the 22 countries from where they came.

The bus trip back to the hotel was even more nerve-wracking in the dark and every time the bus lurched into a loose patch of sand I prayed we would not get bogged. It was after 10pm and everyone was extremely tired and looking forward to enjoying their first night (for most) in a comfortable hotel bed. The last thing we wanted was to get bogged and stranded on a track in the jungle. Fortunately it didn't happen and we made it back to the hotel in time for the first of the leavers to grab their bags and get to the airport in time for their flights.

******

The next morning everyone who was still in Santarem met up in the hotel restaurant for breakfast and continued the conversations from where we had left off the night before. It was a chance to exchange email and Facebook contact details and learn a bit more about each other outside of the Jungle Marathon.

While walking back to my room after breakfast I met up with Shirley and was glad to see that I hadn't missed saying goodbye to her. Everyone was still in the dark about her non-appearance at the dinner the night before and she was very apologetic while explaining that she had been threatened by the villagers in Belterra, where the disqualified runner came from, and that they would "get" her at the finish line or at the party, so she sent them a message saying she would wait to talk to them at the hotel. As soon as the last person had crossed the finish line at Maracana Beach she had gone straight to the hotel and stayed there all day and all evening to see them and avoid any potential dramas at the party. She didn't want runners to have a final memory of a drama at the presentation party.

Shirley continued to explain how she had briefed her staff and sent a letter to give to Basti explaining what she was doing and asked that he make a quick announcement and distribute the prizes. It wasn't known if the message actually got to Basti. She had also sent an email to all the runners explaining and apologizing for her absence but very few people would have had mobile devices on them so no one would have got the message until possibly days later when they were back in their home countries.

While the rest of us were out enjoying the great food and company it seems that Shirley had spent the evening in her hotel room with just a pizza and a glass of wine to keep her company. It was certainly not the way she had hoped to be celebrating the closing moments of the 9th Jungle Marathon.

Considering how heavily Shirley relied on the local people to help her with the logistics of running the event she was concerned about how the events of the past few days would affect future running's of the Jungle Marathon. It would certainly be a shame to have to call an end to the event, especially with 2014 bringing the 10th anniversary of the world's toughest endurance race. For now though, she was just hoping to get home safely and put all of this behind her.

The rest of the day was spent saying goodbye to everyone as we all went our separate ways on different flights staggered throughout the day. I had 6 flights ahead of me and I wasn't looking forward to the 36 hours of travelling to get home, but I guess that would be the final test of endurance in my Jungle Marathon adventure!

Chapter 12

JUNGLE MARATHON CONCLUSION

The Jungle Marathon was not just an endurance race but an epic adventure. This event "raised the bar" so high on my scale of achievements that I'm sure it will be a long time – *if ever* – before I surpass it. The test of strength, endurance and tenacity was punctuated by inspiring moments of appreciation for the beauty of the mighty Amazon Jungle. It is impossible to compare this event to any other because there simply is nothing like it!

I not only pushed myself to limits I didn't even know I could reach but did it in the company of an incredibly inspiring group of amazing athletes and the friendliest volunteers you could possibly hope for. Everyone involved made it an adventure of a lifetime that I will never forget.

Lessons Learnt

* There is a HUGE difference between doing a single day trail marathon and a multiday ultra-endurance marathon!

* If I wasn't already sure of it before, then I'm definitely sure of it now – I hate camping.

* I hate dehydrated meals. While no one else seemed to have a problem with them I loathed them. I will definitely have to investigate other sources of nutrition if I ever forget how much pain I was in at the Jungle Marathon and register for another multi-stage ultra-endurance race.

Things I Regret Not Doing…

* Speaking to more of the competitors and volunteers and getting to hear their story. While writing this book I realized how few people I really spoke to and many of the names in the results table I couldn't even put a face to. I hate that. To the amazing women who completed the 127km event I apologize for not taking the time to congratulate you on your amazing achievements although in my defense, you were so far ahead of me that I don't think I ever saw you! Andreia and Stephanie, you are incredible athletes and your finishing times for each stage reflect the world class competitors this race attracts. All the other women were also great competitors but I'm especially in awe of the four female finishers in the 254km event – you are legends to have survived that!

* Thanking the race volunteers for all their support. I'm afraid by the end of Stage 1 I was too wrecked at the end of each day to say much at all so I hope you all understand now that I was not being rude but just too exhausted to do anything but lie in my hammock.

* Keeping my camera with me so I could take photos along the route. The giant bamboo, the furry caterpillars, the big spiders, the amazing swamps, the beautiful fluvial beaches – but most of all, the people. I'm so grateful for Alexander Beer's photos from the key moments in the race.

* Making an effort to communicate with the many Brazilian and other non-English speaking competitors. Congratulations to you all on your amazing achievements.

Special Mentions

* A big thank you to Shirley for providing me with an alternative backpack when I realized mine wasn't going to be big enough. I repaid the favor to Themos by passing my pack onto him so he could upgrade from the one day marathon to the four day 127km event. There were also many other occasions where people shared gear, helped mend shoes and provided assistance and companionship to runners who were found in need of help. The camaraderie amongst competitors was amazing and injured runners were always taken care of by fellow runners who came across them on the track.

* Winner of the wet T-shirt competition goes to Gustavo Rodrigues and many thanks to UVU for providing the outstanding hot climate racing gear. Basti Haag had almost talked me into buying the same clothes months before the race so I am now extremely grateful he didn't have my size! I'm sure the race photographers would have been very happy if the women were all wearing the same shirts at the checkpoint wash down area. My biggest regret is that I was so far behind Gustavo that his shirt had well and truly dried by the time I caught up to him in the camp each night. Thanks again to Alexander Beer for immortalizing the moment.

JUNGLE MARATHON CONCLUSION

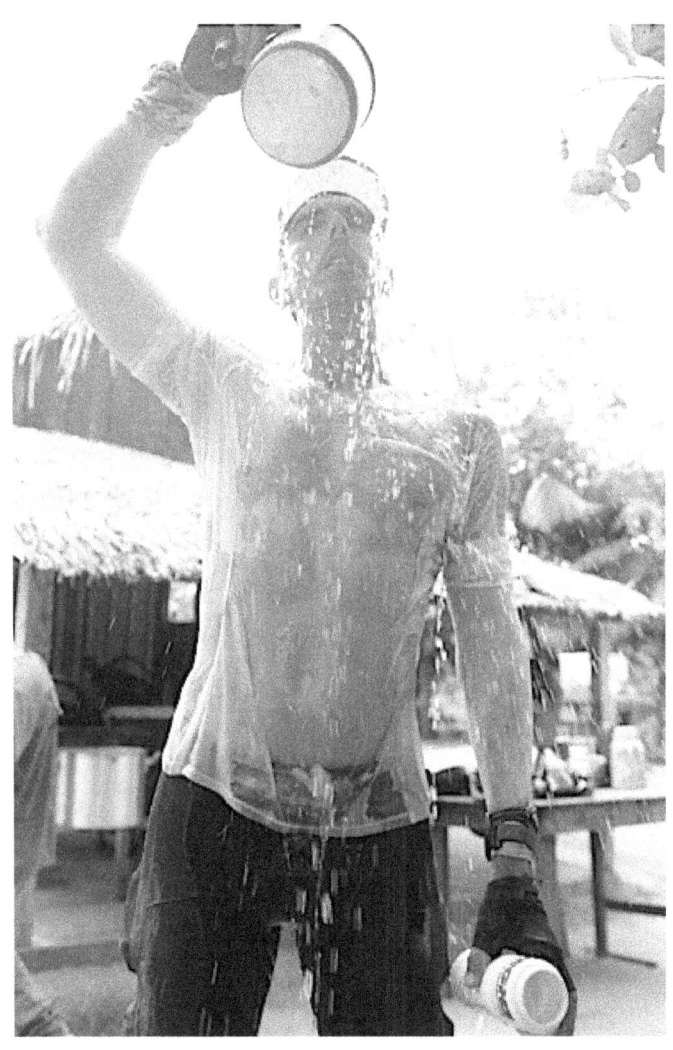

The 2013 Jungle Marathon Comes To An End

Despite the drama that unfolded in the final stages of the 2013 Jungle Marathon - or maybe it's *because* of the drama – Shirley will be preparing to make the 10th anniversary edition of the Jungle Marathon in 2014 live up to it's reputation of being the toughest endurance race in the world. Being an ultra-endurance runner herself, Shirley isn't about to let a few hiccups get in the way of continuing an event that every adventurous endurance runner should have on their bucket list.

If you want to be a part of the toughest race in the world - in the most amazing place in the world - then the Jungle Marathon is for you!

EPILOGUE

After all the training and preparation, the Jungle Marathon is now just an amazing memory of an adventure in the remote Amazon Jungle with an incredible group of people. To say it lived up to my expectations is an understatement – *it was much harder than I could ever have imagined!*

The 2013 Jungle Marathon proved to be challenging not only for the competitors but also for the race director. An unexpected turn of events resulting from action taken to discourage cheating, forced the race organizers to re-evaluate the course for future events and plan to avoid regions that lie outside the national park boundaries, where they have less control. While the safety of the runners is paramount, it is impossible to eliminate every possible risk in such an extreme environment, and it's these inherent risks that add to the excitement and drive adventurous athletes to such events.

2014 will see the 10th anniversary running of the Jungle Marathon with another group of ultra-endurance athletes participating in the world's most extreme endurance race.

The Jungle Marathon is a must-do for every endurance athlete who is after not only the ultimate physical challenge but also the experience of a lifetime.

JUNGLE MARATHON 2013 RESULTS

254km 6-Stage Event - MALE

Pos	Athlete	Race No	Country	Total Time
1	Marcelo Sinoca	35	Brazil	32:18:14
2	Rodrigo Souza	36	Brazil	34:21:02
3	Sebastian Haag	14	Germany	35:33:50
4	Gustavo Rodrigues	76	Brazil	37:49:54
5	Jean-Paul Van Der Bas	78	Netherlands	39:12:03
6	Mario Angel Oyola	25	Argentina	39:34:37
7	Krzysztof Sobczak	37	Poland	40:13:42
8	Jason Wolfe	44	USA	40:29:00
9	Alex Vicintin	43	Brazil	40:29:25
10	Roberto Ameiro	1	Brazil	42:04:07
11	Eder Morimoto	75	Brazil	43:53:06
12	Jerlison Almeida	73	Brazil	43:57:46
13	Regis Botter	4	Brazil	44:40:57
14	Geovane Rento de Carvalho	30	Brazil	46:01:47
15	Lien Choong Luen	20	Singapore	46:11:57
16	Anthony Hugill	15	UK	47:08:18
17	Marcelo Vanzuita	47	NZ	47:54:00
18	Moon-Ka Leung	19	China	50:48:12
19	Ricardo da Silva	8	Brazil	51:15:39
20	Alfredo DiMeo	9	UK	52:18:27
21	Pedro Jimenez	16	Venezuela	52:43:55
22	Matt Buck	6	USA	52:43:31

23	Jereon Roodenburg	33	Netherlands	53:08:43
24	Petter Vallestad	49	Norway	55:55:17
25	Berndt Tvedt	70	Norway	55:55:31
26	Cleber Evangelista	71	Brazil	56:33:54
27	Antonio Giannella	13	Italy	62:24:17
Completed Less Than 4 Stages				
	Vinicius Boscolo	5	Brazil	Stage 1,2,3
	Yoshizo Yokoyama	45	Japan	Stages 1,2,6
	Luis Menendez	23	Argentina	Stage 1

254km 6-Stage Event - FEMALE

Pos	Athlete	Race No	Country	Total Time
1	Jacqueline Terto	38	Brazil	45:55:33
2	Marie Danet	7	France	57:40:43
3	Kim Frankish	12	UK	74:32:48
4	Jacquie Palmer	24	USA	76:07:28

127km 4-Stage Event - MALE

Pos	Athlete	Race No	Country	Total Time
1	Lucas Marques	22	Brazil	18:55:09
2	Themos Sgouras	61	Greece	24:21:03
3	Clayton Conservani	40	Brazil	26:25:03
4	Mike Kraft	17	Germany	26:51:07
5	Mauricio Gomes	57	Brazil	27:23:24
6	Michael Ford	11	UK	28:30:16
7	Ed Burns	48	UK	33:17:36
8	Jason Schneider	52	USA	33:29:38
9	Henrique Pina	28	Brazil	35:42:37
254km Competitors who dropped down to 127km				
	Bernard Plessberger	29	Austria	15:22:31
	Hirofumi Ono	72	Japan	19:58:22
	Sergio Retamales	63	Chile	31:19:52
	Michael Assenmacher	2	Germany	33:49:38

127km 4-Stage Event - FEMALE

Pos	Athlete	Race No	Country	Total Time
1	Andreia Henssler	51	Brazil	23:05:56
2	Stefanie Bacon	46	UK	23:39:19
3	Carol Barcello	42	Brazil	26:24:58
4	Anna Chernova	79	Switzerland	27:10:14
5	Danielle Whitney	67	USA	33:22:48
6	Karen Curtis	50	Australia	33:29:42
254km Competitors who dropped down to 127km				
	Amanda Barlow	3	Australia	32:46:28

42km – Marathon Stage – MALE and FEMALE

Pos	Athlete	Race No	Country	Total Time
1	Orlando de Sousa Patrocino	41	Brazil	4:52:56
2	Leandro Ribeiro Vaz	84	Brazil	5:20:24
3	Marcelo Alves	69	Brazil	5:30:37
4	Gercilson dos Santos	62	Brazil	8:08:41
5	*Alaene dos Santos*	*66*	*Brazil*	*8:37:16*
6	Manoel Joao de Sousa Moreira	59	Brazil	9:11:16
7	Kelven Mota da Silva	85	Brazil	9:11:25
8	Aurelio Luciano	10	Brazil	9:22:18
9	Luiz Lacerda	39	Brazil	9:26:55
10	Joao Carlos Pijnappel	74	Brazil	9:55:22
11	Sebastian Armenault	42	Argentina	13:39:10
254km Competitors who dropped down to Marathon				
	Lee Morris	77	Wales	8:16:00
	Luis Menendez	23	Argentina	10:46:11
	Fredrick Lowestetter	80	USA	14:22:01
	Sandra Simons	*66*	*USA*	*14:22:02*

CALL OF THE JUNGLE

ABOUT THE AUTHOR

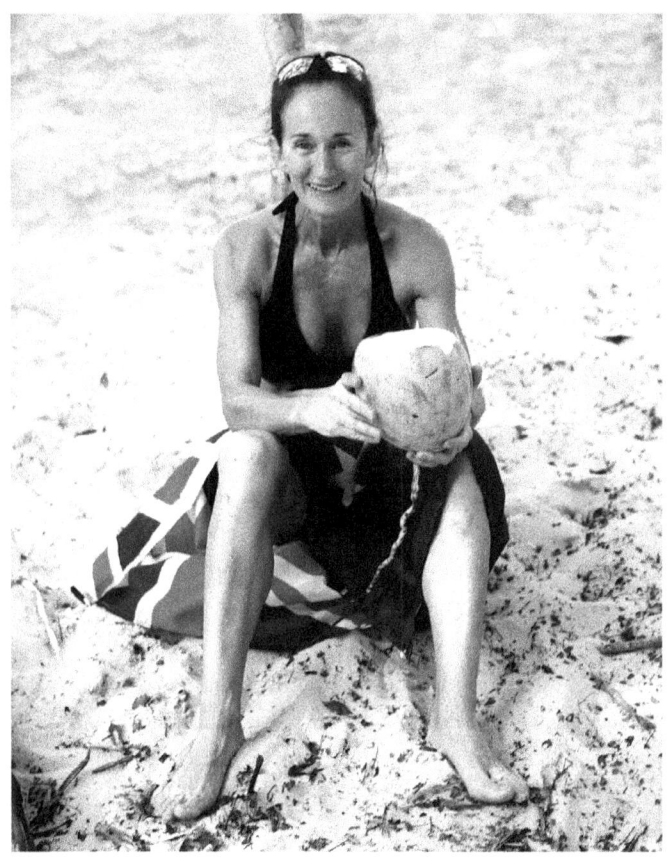

Amanda Barlow is a recreational marathon runner who ran her first marathon in 2009, at the age of 49, at the London Marathon. Since then she has completed marathons on all seven continents, earning her an entry into the Seven Continents Marathon Club in November 2012, after running the following marathons: London and Gold Coast 2009, Barcelona and Marine Corps Marathon (Washington DC) 2011, Kilimanjaro Marathon (Tanzania), Great Wall Marathon (China), Inca Trail Marathon (Peru), and finally the Antarctic Ice Marathon in 2012.

Prior to competing in the Jungle Marathon in October 2013, Amanda had run over 16 marathons, including the ill-fated 2013 Boston Marathon.

The 54-year old mother of three adult children works as a Wellsite Geologist on offshore oil and gas rigs and subsequently is confined to doing most of her training on a treadmill, or running round in circles on a helideck. While the 360° ocean views from the helideck are a peaceful backdrop for running, the repetitive tight circles can cause dizziness and one leg to become shorter than the other so her preference for longer runs is on the treadmill.

Competing in "destination" marathons is Amanda's idea of a holiday, and with many more of the worlds natural wonders to explore, there will no doubt be many more marathons yet to run. The wonderful people she has met, and new friends she has made, have helped fuel her passion for keeping fit so she can continue to run around the world – *literally*!

www.ingramcontent.com/pod-product-compliance
Lightning Source LLC
Chambersburg PA
CBHW070547050426
42450CB00011B/2759